EPIDEMIOLOGY, BEHAVIOR CHANGE, AND INTERVENTION IN CHRONIC DISEASE

EPIDEMIOLOGY, BEHAVIOR CHANGE, AND INTERVENTION IN CHRONIC DISEASE

Edited by

Linda K. Hall, PhD
The Christ Hospital

G. Curt Meyer, MS
Lee Memorial Hospital

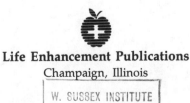

Life Enhancement Publications
Champaign, Illinois

Library of Congress Cataloging-in-Publication Data

Epidemiology, behavior change, and intervention in
    chronic disease.
    (La Crosse exercise and health series)
    Includes bibliographies.
    1. Chronically ill—Rehabilitation—Psychological
aspects. 2. Patient compliance. 3. Exercise therapy.
4. Diabetes—Rehabilitation—Psychological aspects.
5. Chronic obstructive pulmonary disease—Patients—
Rehabilitation—Psychological aspects. I. Hall,
Linda K. II. Meyer, G. Curt. III. Series.
RC108.E65   1988   616   87-26185
ISBN 0-87322-912-6

Developmental Editor: Lisa Busjahn
Production Director: Ernie Noa
Projects Manager: Lezli Harris
Copy Editor: Peter Nelson
Assistant Editor: Julie Anderson
Typesetter: Yvonne Winsor
Text Design: Keith Blomberg
Text Layout: Denise Peters
Printed By: Braun-Brumfield, Inc.

ISBN: 0-87322-912-6
ISSN: 0894-4261

Printed in the United States of America

10 9 8 7 6 5 4 3 2 1

Life Enhancement Publications
A Division of Human Kinetics Publishers, Inc.
Box 5076, Champaign, IL 61820
1-800-342-5457
1-800-334-3665 (in Illinois)

Contributors

Barbara N. Campaigne Lipid Research Clinic, Cincinnati, Ohio

Gerilynn Connors Pulmonary Rehabilitation Center, St. Helena Health Center, Deer Park, California

Jerry A. Dempsey, PhD John Rankin Laboratory of Pulmonary Medicine, University of Wisconsin, Madison, Wisconsin

Rod K. Dishman, PhD Director, Behavioral Fitness Laboratory, University of Georgia, Athens, Georgia

Debra Dodson Drake, MS Feelin' Good Fitness Center, Spring Arbor, Michigan

Linda K. Hall, PhD Director, Cardiac Rehabilitation Center, The Christ Hospital, Cincinnati, Ohio

Kathe G. Henke John Rankin Laboratory of Pulmonary Medicine, University of Wisconsin, Madison, Wisconsin

Charles T. Kuntzleman, EdD Feelin' Good Fitness Center, Spring Arbor, Michigan

Ralph S. Paffenbarger, Jr., MD Stanford University School of Medicine, Stanford, California

Catherine Reith Murphy, MS American Rehabilitation Center, Camp Hill, Pennsylvania

Marge Samsoe, MS Cardiac Rehabilitation Center, Gunderson Clinic, La Crosse, Wisconsin

James W. Terman, MD Department of Internal Medicine, Gunderson Clinic—Lutheran Hospital, La Crosse, Wisconsin

Contents

Series Preface

On behalf of the chapter authors and editors and Human Kinetics Publishers, it is my pleasure to welcome you to this book. *Epidemiology, Behavior Change, and Intervention in Chronic Disease* is one of a collection of eight books of the La Crosse Exercise and Health Series, offered by Life Enhancement Publications of Human Kinetics Publishers. The series is an outgrowth of various topics of the annual symposiums of the La Crosse Exercise and Health Program of the University of Wisconsin-La Crosse. Offered by the program's Educational Services Unit, these symposiums are directed to professionals in athletic training and rehabilitation, cardiac rehabilitation, corporate and hospital-based fitness and wellness programs, nutrition, and sports medicine. The individual editors of each book in the series were initially responsible for developing the topics and presenters for that specific symposium.

We intend for these books to provide readers with both theoretical and practical information specific to their fields of interest. Symposium topics and speakers, and consequently chapter authors, have been chosen to provide "hands-on" information to assist practitioners. The symposiums and the resulting books are intended to truly assist you in the everyday practice of your profession. Cognitive knowledge applied in both theory and practice to daily problems and concerns is the ultimate goal of the La Crosse symposiums and book series. It is truly the hope of the symposium presenters and chapter authors, of the book editors, and of myself that each reader finds the information provided appropriately serves their daily professional needs.

On behalf of the chapter authors and book editors, I thank Human Kinetics Publishers of Champaign, Illinois, for its involvement as the La Crosse Series publisher. Over the past 10 years Human Kinetics has become a leading publisher in the field of health and physical fitness, and we are pleased and appreciative for its commitment to this book series.

Philip K. Wilson, EdD
Series Editor

Preface

This book is divided into two sections: (1) a comprehensive look at epidemiological perspectives in disease, behavioral change, and motivation, and (2) an examination of exercise testing, education, and exercise prescription for the general public and the chronically ill. As more people adopt the wellness outlook it becomes clearer that poor health knowledge and learned risk behaviors account for more disease onset and premature deaths than any other factors. Ninety-eight percent of all babies born today are healthy; with the control of the formerly dreaded childhood diseases polio, pneumonia, and tuberculosis, they have an average life span of approximately 78 years (National Center for Health Promotion, 1986).

Recent research at the Carter Center at Emory University in Atlanta, Georgia, has found that ignorance and learned behavior result in 14 major factors responsible for 85% of health care expenditures and 80% of deaths, with 8.5 million life-years lost each year (University of California, 1986). (A life-year is defined as each year of life lost as a result of dying before the age of 65. For example, if a person dies at age 55, 10 life-years are lost.) This study considers death before age of 65 as premature and recommends prevention and education as "magic bullets" for cutting health care costs and preventing disabling diseases and premature deaths.

Studies Indicate Decline in Fitness Levels

Recent survey results of the President's Council on Physical Fitness and Sports (PCPFS) show that there has been no recent improvement in fitness when today's young people are compared to their counterparts of 1958 (Murphy, 1986). (What's worse, it was the poor fitness of those youths in 1958 when compared to European youths that led President Eisenhower to establish the PCPFS.) The survey results further show that in some ways there have been declines in fitness levels.

Many reasons can be cited for the poor fitness of American children: television and other video diversions with estimated monthly averages of 39 hours of viewing time but only 11 hours of physical activity; increased mechanization, with stairs replaced by elevators and walking by car rides; budget cuts causing the cessation of physical education courses in many schools; and a strong tendency to be spectators rather than participants (Brataas, 1986).

A major factor to consider is whether organized children's sports indeed promote fitness. It can be easy to believe that because children are involved in "little league" football, baseball, basketball, hockey, and soccer, they are getting activity intense enough and of sufficient duration to produce cardiorespiratory fitness. However, Pat Shibinski of the College of Mount St. Joseph has noted that "there is an awful lot of sitting and standing around in many team sports." Connie Kampschmidt of the University of Cincinnati adds that if you don't make the team, you go home and sit, and that's where poor fitness begins (Brataas, 1986).

Poor health habits, especially concerning exercise and nutrition, begin taking their toll in childhood and can be precursors to chronic diseases that manifest themselves as children grow into adulthood. A recent study in the *New England Journal of Medicine* (Newman et al., 1986) has presented evidence that heart disease begins early in life. Autopsies of 35 people between the ages of 11 and 23, who had died of causes other than heart disease, showed that 6 of them had coronary artery fatty deposits equal to those found in adults. The director of the study, Dr. Gerald Berenson of the Louisiana State University Medical Center, thinks health education and illness prevention should begin in childhood. Chapter 4 in this book looks at the prevention efforts of the Fitness Finders program in Spring Arbor, Michigan. Their results show that through education and family and school commitment, changes in children's risk factors can be made (Drake, 1987).

Obesity's Relation to Chronic Illness

Obesity is a growing problem among today's young people. An estimated one-third of children and teenagers under the age of 18 are obese (obesity is defined here as when fat comprises more than 30% of total body weight). Much research has indicated that while obesity is not a direct cause of many of today's chronic diseases, it certainly can exacerbate them. Sharon Hoerr (1984) has found that few Type II diabetics are not obese; few obese people do not have high cholesterol levels, and one in three teenage girls is on a diet, which more often than not is dangerous. One of the 19-year-old patients in the eating disorders unit at The Christ Hospital was an infancy onset diabetic who found she could be thin by not taking her insulin and by supplementing her daily output by stealing and ingesting her father's diuretics. (She also discovered that she could become very sick.) Hoerr has contended that there is a social stigma against overweight among adolescent girls, exacerbated by the model of beauty pushed in the media.

Recent studies have shown that though the predisposition to obesity is largely genetically controlled, and that though nothing can be done to prevent the transmission of the genetic coding allowing varying degrees of fatness, there are methods available to insure that obesity does not necessarily result. Albert Stunkard and co-workers have suggested defensive eating and a high degree of activity to thwart obesity genes ("Genetics Important," 1986; Stunkard et al., 1986). Several studies have concurred with Stunkard and have demonstrated that with increased endurance activities, such as aerobic exercise, there is a decrease or only a very slight increase in food intake, creating a negative energy balance, resulting in fat weight loss (Epstein, Masek, & Marshall, 1978; Holm, Bjorntrop, & Jagenburg, 1978; Woo, Garrow, & Pi-Sunger, 1981). There is also evidence that activity reduces both the size and number of fat cells (Askew & Heckner, 1976; Oscai et al., 1972, 1974).

The Importance of Behavioral Change

All of the preceding information has been devoted to the prepubescent and adolescent. Usually behavior patterns are established in early childhood during the first 10-12 formative years. This points up the importance environment has in establishing behaviors that can greatly affect health. Statistics can be cited with regard to the high incidence of smoking, drinking, and obesity in children of smoking, drinking, and obese parents ("Education Useful," 1986; Gannett News Service, 1986; Klein, 1986). The hereditary role in heart disease is well known, yet, environmental risk factors (e.g., smoking, high cholesterol diets, a lack of regular exercise) generally enhance the likelihood of heart disease.

Environment and behavior are the two major influences in chronic disease and premature death. Unfortunately, once behavior has been programmed, it usually takes a major event such as a heart attack, bypass surgery, or cancer to initiate change. Some in the rehabilitation field even find patients who feel it is too late to change and continue harmful behavior, hastening death. Those who do change often become healthier and live better than they had for a long time. Others, no matter the amount of changes made, still do not change the final outcome.

There are many theories behind the development of methods for initiating behavior change. No matter which method is chosen, there are certain components necessary for it to work:

- A healthy self-esteem
- An acceptance of your situation
- An awareness of the positive behavior needed
- Information on the behavior
- The formulation of a plan
- Skills necessary for the change
- Intrinsic and extrinsic motivation
- A positive support system
- The change is not viewed as a punishment and has achievable goals (Edington, 1986; O'Donnell, 1986).

A behavior change program must become a family affair. If one person in a family is trying to quit smoking, for example, but all others in the household continue to smoke, the behavior change is nearly impossible. It is hoped that when one in the family makes a decision to change, discussion and contracting to establish a "change-enhancing environment" by all family members will occur. When disease strikes a parent and risk factor control or elimination becomes necessary, the modified behavior will ripple throughout the whole family, precluding the disease from striking generations to come ("Behavior Change," 1986; "Health Education," 1985).

This book holds a holistic approach to health and behavior. The first section examines epidemiological precursors to disease, methods with children, and motivation. The second section discusses exercise testing, exercise prescription, and education in chronic diseases, using the cardiac rehabilitation model. This book will certainly enhance the practical background of professionals in the field of rehabilitation and health intervention.

Linda K. Hall

References

Askew, E.W., & Hecker, A.L. (1976). Adipose tissue cell size and lipolysis in the rat: Response to exercise intensity and food restriction. *Journal of Nutrition*, **106**, 1351-1360.

Brataas, A. (1986). Nation's babies are sitters. *Cincinnati Enquirer.*

Drake, D. (1987). Early intervention/prevention in childhood. In L.K. Hall, G.C. Meyer, & P.J. Paffenbarger (Eds.), *Epidemiology, behavior change, and intervention in chronic disease.* Champaign, IL: Human Kinetics.

Edington, D.W. (1986, May/June). Research update: Health behaviors tied to education level. *Optimal Health*, p. 60.

Epstein, L., Masek, B., & Marshall, W. (1978). Nutritionally based school program for control of eating in obese children. *Behavior Therapy, 9,* 766-788.

Gannet News Service. (1986, August 31). Study links heart attacks, smoking. *Cincinnati Enquirer.*

Genetics important factor in body weight, study says. (1986, January 23). *Washington Post.*

Health education/risk reduction: Helping healthy children stay healthy. (1985, November). *Momentum Toward Health,* HHS-NIH, p. 62.

Hoerr, S.L. (1984). Exercise: An alternative to fad diets for adolescent girls. *The Physician and Sportsmedicine, 12,* 76-83.

Holm, G., Bjorntrop, P., & Jagenburg, R. (1978). Carbohydrate, lipid, and amino acid metabolism following physical exercise in man. *Journal of Applied Physiology, 45,* 128-131.

Klein, J. (1986, October). Firsthand look at secondhand risk. *American Health,* p. 14.

Murphy, P. (1986). Youth fitness testing: A matter of health or performance. *The Physician and Sportsmedicine, 14,* 189-190.

National Center for Health Promotion. (1986, Winter/Spring). *Health notes.* Ann Arbor, Michigan.

Newman, W.P., Freedman, D.S., & Voors, A.W. (1986). Relation of serum lipoprotein levels and systolic blood pressure to early atherosclerosis: The Bogalusa heart study. *New England Journal of Medicine, 314,* 138-143.

O'Donnell, M.P. (1986). Design of workplace health promotion programs. *American Journal of Health Promotion.*

Oscai, L.B., Babirak, S.P., & McGarr, J.A. (1974). Effect of exercise on adipose tissue cellularity. *Federation Proceedings, 33,* 1956-1958.

Oscai, L.B., Spirakis, C.N., & Wolff, C.A. (1972). Effects of exercise and food restriction on adipose tissue cellularity. *Journal of Lipid Research, 13,* 588-592.

Staff. (1986, April 28). Education useful in cutting heart risk factors. *AMA News.*

Staff. (1986, July/August). Behavior change, it's still the biggest challenge. *Optimal Health,* pp. 24-28.

Staff. (1986, February). The magic bullet is prevention. *University of California Berkeley Wellness Letter,* p. 1.

Stunkard, A.J., Sorensen, T.I., Hanis, C., & Teasdale, T.W. (1986). An adoption study of human obesity. *New England Journal of Medicine, 314,* 193-198.

Woo, R., Garrow, J., & Pi-Sunger, F. (1981). Effect of exercise on spontaneous calorie intake in obesity, abstracted. *Clinical Research, 29,* 621.

Part I

Epidemiology, Behavior Change, and Adherence

Chapter 1

Epidemiologic Perspectives of Exercise and Behavioral Management in the Prevention of Chronic Disease

Ralph S. Paffenbarger, Jr.

By identifying frequency distributions, determinants, and deterrents of disease in human populations, epidemiologic methods provide the principal means to evaluate the roles of physical activity and personal behaviors in the cause and prevention of chronic disease. The literature contains a variety of epidemiologic studies of physical activity, exploring personal athleticism and less energetic activities as a first line of defense against coronary heart disease (CHD) and other chronic diseases.

Writers of antiquity, employing techniques of comparison common to modern epidemiologic methods, observed from the disease experiences of population clusters that a sedentary lifestyle and overeating were detrimental to health. Attention to the value of exercise is as old as Hippocrates, whose remarks on the hazards of physical inactivity were cited by Bernardino Ramazzini in 1700, along with comments on dangers of athletic overstress. Ramazzini (1964) contrasted the health of sedentary tailors with physically active "runners," or messengers. Both low and high extremes of exertion were unwise, inviting ill effects, he said. Because tailors could not expect to get enough physical activity at work, "they should be advised to take physical exercise at any rate on holidays. Let them make the best use they can of some one day, and so to counteract the harm done by many days of sedentary life." Today health professionals offer this same advice to the millions of workers from whom energy-saving devices, electronics, and robots have removed much opportunity for strenuous physical output on the job.

Today in societies where infectious diseases are largely under control, except where AIDS-related diseases will take an enormous toll, the focus is ever more sharply on the study and prevention of chronic disease. Behavioral management is receiving intensified attention for practical intervention strategies, such as adjustment of exercise levels and other patterns of living influencing health. This is illustrated in Table 1, which is taken from epidemiologic observations on a group of college alumni whose cause-specific death rates are presented in relation to given levels of energy expenditure in walking, stair climbing, and sports play (Paffenbarger, Hyde, Wing, & Steinmetz, 1984). In this population cardiovascular and respiratory diseases account for approximately half of all deaths, and their rates are strongly associated with physical activity level. Although other elements of lifestyle also affect risk of these diseases, adequate exercise patterns would seem to be highly important as a means of avoiding or postponing deaths from such causes. In contrast, exercise is not

Table 1   Cause-Specific Death Rates per 10,000 Man-Years of Observation Among 16,936 Harvard Alumni, 1962-78, by Physical Activity Index

Cause of Death (n)	Physical Activity Index (kcal/week)			One-tail test for trend, p
	< 500	500-1,999	2,000+	
All causes (1,413)	84.8	66.0	52.1	< .001
Total cardiovascular diseases (640)	39.5	30.8	21.4	< .001
Coronary heart disease (441)	25.7	21.2	16.4	.002
Stroke (103)	6.5	5.2	2.4	.001
Total respiratory diseases (60)	6.0	3.2	1.5	.001
Total cancers (446)	25.7	19.2	19.0	.026
Lung (89)	6.2	3.7	4.0	.116
Colorectal (58)	2.2	2.3	3.5	.091*
Pancreas (41)	1.8	2.4	1.0	.085
Prostate (36)	2.2	1.5	1.6	.359
Total unnatural causes (146)	8.7	7.1	5.9	.032
Accidents (78)	3.6	3.9	3.0	.147
Suicides (68)	5.1	3.2	2.9	.049

Note. Adjusted for differences in age, cigarette smoking, and hypertension. From "A Natural History of Athleticism and Cardiovascular Health" by R.S. Paffenbarger, Jr., R.T. Hyde, A.L. Wing, and C.H. Steinmetz, 1984, *Journal of the American Medical Association*, **252**(4), p. 494. Copyright 1984, American Medical Association.

*Opposite trend.

a predominant influence on cancer mortality, and the discouragement of cigarette smoking or correction of overeating may have greater control there, although such actions are important in the control of cardio-respiratory diseases, also. With these points as a starting place, a review of the progress in studying the epidemiologic aspects of cardiovascular diseases should be of interest.

Since 1950 many studies have shown that adequate physical exercise should have high prospects as an intervention regimen against CHD. Though demands for strenuous physical activity on the job have been disappearing, leisure-time exercise, such as vigorous sports play, has become more frequent. In the more developed countries, a boom in highly active recreational pursuits has greatly altered the lifestyles of young and old in large segments of the population.

Energy expenditure is inversely related to incidence of nonfatal and fatal CHD, and this association is at least partly independent of other influences (Morris et al., 1973; Morris, Everitt, Pollard, Chave, & Semmence, 1980; Paffenbarger, Wing, & Hyde, 1978). Although many studies have confirmed these findings, the complexities of the total lifestyle picture have led to considerable skepticism, much of it probably unwarranted. Unlike obesity, cigarette smoking, hypertension, and several other characteristics known to influence CHD risk, diet and exercise are universal: Everyone must take in and expend energy, whether the amounts are too little, sufficient, or in excess (Wood et al., 1983; Wood, 1983). With so many interacting variables, precisely controlled studies of exercise are difficult to arrange and maintain, and more reliance must be placed on assessing "natural" circumstances by epidemiologic methods. The results of a number of these investigations will be described briefly.

Occupational Physical Activity

Coronary heart disease was first described in 1912, but its inverse relationship to adequate vigorous exercise was not pointed out until J.N. Morris and associates in 1953 described epidemiologic findings on CHD incidence among London busmen (Morris, 1975; Morris, Heady, Raffle, Roberts, & Parks, 1953; Morris, Kagan, Pattison, Gardner, & Raffle, 1966). Physically active conductors, scrambling to collect tickets on double-decked buses, had much lower rates of CHD than the bus drivers, who were sedentary all day.

This report sparked further studies of occupations in many countries because rising CHD incidence had prompted worldwide alarm. Inverse patterns of exercise level and CHD risk were found between letter carriers and mail clerks (Kahn, 1963), farmers and sedentary townsmen (Cassel et al., 1971; Zukel et al., 1959), workers on different jobs in kibbutzim in Israel (Brunner, Manelis, Modan, & Levin, 1974), railroad track workers and clerks (Menotti & Puddu, 1976; Taylor et al., 1962), and San Francisco longshoremen loading cargo into ship holds or tallying it into warehouses (Paffenbarger, Laughlin, Gima, & Black, 1970). Meanwhile Morris was refining his own work (Morris, 1975).

Even the most persuasive epidemiologic studies drew attention to the problems in assessing exercise and its relationships to other CHD risk factors. Some reports ignored exercise, partly because such other influences as diet, cigarette smoking, and blood lipid levels were receiving new attention. Also, populations differed in lifestyles, and there were wide departures in availability of data and methods of analysis. Perhaps more importantly, many studies (and questionnaires) were not designed principally to test the exercise-CHD hypothesis, and "afterthought analyses" often were based on types and amounts of physical activity that were inadequately assessed. Findings were negative among civil service employees in Los Angeles (Chapman & Massey, 1964) and Chicago industrial workers (Paul et al., 1963; Stamler et al., 1960) largely because the job categories lacked contrast in physical activity demands, and leisure-time energy output had not been studied. Ethnic and cultural differences apparently compounded such problems when a complex 10-year study was attempted of 16 demographic cohorts in seven countries (Keys, 1980). A four-part question related to occupational activities distinguished groups at low and high CHD risk in only half of the cohorts.

Whether exercise levels range from sedentariness to high energy output, no matter in what pattern, and even if its contributions are masked from study by such other elements of lifestyle as diet and leisure-time activities, exercise is universally present and influential in all populations. When interacting characteristics are inadequately defined and considered, conclusions drawn from analysis may become contradictory or confused. In some cases inconclusive findings as to exercise and CHD risk have been refuted by subsequent studies of the same populations or extended analyses of later data (Karvonen, 1981, 1982; Salonen, Puska, & Tuomilehto, 1982). As various predictors of CHD, such as blood fractions of lipoprotein-cholesterol, have become better understood, epidemiologic study design, data-gathering instruments, trend sampling, coding, data processing, evaluation, and interpretation of results have been refined.

The San Francisco Longshoremen Study

Following multiphasic screening examinations in 1951, nearly 4,000 San Francisco stevedores were followed for 22 years to assess their work activity and fatal CHD levels. Exercise patterns were assessed by on-the-job energy output measurements. Shifts in job assignments were checked annually, occupational exercise was noted in kilocalories per week

(Kcal/week), and mortality rates were derived from official death certificates and man-years of observation. Cargohandlers loading and unloading ships contrasted strongly with foremen and clerks lodged in sedentary assignments. Unsturdy men were unlikely to be found in either group, as union rules required all members to be cargohandlers for at least their first 5 years of employment. Most did heavy work much longer, 13 years on average, and shifted to less physically demanding jobs not for health reasons but for reasons of higher pay and prestige. These work practices suggest that the differing CHD rates for longshoremen in high and low energy-output jobs could not be accounted for by hereditary self-selection alone, nor by adjustment for job transfers that might have accompanied premonitory symptoms of impending heart problems (Paffenbarger, 1977; Paffenbarger & Hale, 1975; Paffenbarger, Hale, Brand, & Hyde, 1977).

Death rates of CHD among 3,686 longshoremen from 1951 to 1972 were computed per 10,000 man-years of work, by age at death, and by job energy output category. A total of 395 CHD deaths (11%) occurred during the follow-up, but the rate for cargohandlers who expended 8,500+ Kcal/week at work (32% of the man-years of the follow-up) was only about half (56%) of the rate for men in less demanding jobs. This reduced mortality was greatest at younger ages but evident at all ages. Because the longshoremen usually worked hard in a waterfront occupation all their lives, the findings are especially pertinent. A preliminary study showed that their leisure-time exercise was of relatively little importance alongside their exceptionally high occupational energy output (Paffenbarger & Hale, 1975). Shifting trends and patterns, such as those brought by changes in technology, are among several reasons why for the four 10-year cohorts born between 1877 and 1916, vigorous exercise at work was associated with significantly lower fatal CHD rates only in the two younger cohorts (Paffenbarger, Hale, Brand, & Hyde, 1977).

Cargohandlers had much lower risk of sudden death from CHD than more sedentary fellows. Data on nonfatal CHD were lacking, but the cargohandlers may have been less likely to have an attack or better able to withstand one. The sudden death findings are of further interest if they imply less likelihood that overt premonitory symptoms had induced a change to lighter work assignments, thus detracting from an explanation of self-selection (Brand, Paffenbarger, Sholtz, & Kampert, 1979; Paffenbarger, 1977; Paffenbarger, Brand, Sholtz, & Jung, 1978). Allowing for job transfers during the follow-up period did not appreciably alter the findings for any CHD mortality categories, sudden or delayed. Eliminating the influences of age, cigarette smoking, obesity, high blood pressure, and prior CHD showed a progressive lowering of fatal CHD risk among longshoremen as energy output on the job rose from 4,750 to 10,750 Kcal/week. Risk was reduced by half when energy output doubled above the baseline level.

Leisure-Time Physical Activity

The impact of leisure-time activity on CHD has been examined in various studies. These studies and results will be considered here.

The British Civil Service Study

J.N. Morris and his colleagues saw that leisure-time exercise could influence CHD risk among workers whose sedentary jobs did not afford adequate energy output. They studied a population of 17,944 middle-aged male British civil servants who submitted a standard diary form that logged their physical activities of one work day and the consecutive leisure day. In 8.5 years of follow-up, those who had reported vigorous leisure exercise, such as sports activity, had a CHD rate of 3.1% versus 6.9% for men lacking vigorous exercise. Rates of fatal first-CHD attack for these groups were 1.1 and 2.9%, respectively, and for sudden deaths (unheralded by advance sick leave) 0.65 and 1.60%. Retired civil servants differed likewise. Most importantly, the rise in CHD morbidity with age was prominent only among the nonvigorous groups; there was relatively little increase with age among men who had reported habitual vigorous exercise (usually sports play) (Chave, Morris, Moss, & Semmence, 1978; Epstein, Miller, Stitt, & Morris, 1976; Morris et al., 1973).

As was found for occupational exercise and its influence on CHD risk, the results of epidemiologic investigations of leisure-time physical activity have varied widely. In some, occupational differences may not have been recognized and a presumed similarity would be erroneous. In others, the methods of rating leisure-time exercise may not have been sufficiently refined. A number of recent studies have assessed both occupational and leisure-time physical activity, separately or together, as will be described later.

The U.S. College Alumni Study

An extensive survey of casual and leisure-time exercise among U.S. college alumni is of interest in itself and in comparison with the findings of Morris in England and the longshoremen study in California. Because the college alumni study includes a notably long-range data collection and follow-up, it could provide an exceptional opportunity to study the influences of lifestyle and exercise on CHD risk in the elderly years, on life expectancy, and perhaps on aging. Patterns of leisure-time exercise, other lifestyle elements, and health status among 50,000 former students from Harvard University and the University of Pennsylvania have been under study to determine how past and contemporary physical activity relate to CHD risk (Paffenbarger et al., 1966; Paffenbarger & Wing, 1969;

Paffenbarger, Wolf, Notkin, & Thorne, 1966). Data extending from about 1900 to the present have been obtained from physical examination and other college records of students who matriculated during 1916 through 1950, from alumni responses to self-administered mail questionnaires assessed at several intervals since 1962, and from terminal findings from death certificates. Subsets of the total population have been studied for personal characteristics of college days as well as for present-day exercise habits and physician-diagnosed CHD, using suitable follow-up periods. Analysis has shown that current and continuing adequate exercise, rather than a history of youthful or hereditary vigor and athleticism, is associated inversely with risk of CHD in all age brackets studied. To date there have been approximately 12,000 deaths from all causes, and the surviving alumni are aged 48 to 88 years. The University of Pennsylvania data include 3,500 alumni who entered that college during the years 1931 through 1940, and who currently are being studied by epidemiologic methods for predictive factors of CHD.

Incidence rates of first CHD attack among 16,936 Harvard University alumni during 10 or 6 years (1962 or 1966 to 1972) were calculated per 10,000 man-years, by levels of habitual and leisure-time physical activity. Among 572 stricken alumni aged 35-74, there were 357 nonfatal and 215 fatal first attacks. Age-specific rates of CHD declined consistently with gradient increases in energy expenditure (by stair climbing, walking, and sports play) as determined from mail questionnaires, and likewise with increasing Kcal/week in a composite physical activity index. Similar trends were found for nonfatal and fatal clinical events (angina pectoris, myocardial infarction, and, to a lesser degree, sudden death). Risk patterns of CHD were similar by 10-year age classes from 35 through 74 years. The cardiovascular benefit of continuing adequate exercise held good over a wide range of lifestyles. The benefit of current exercise was heightened by vigorous sports play; specifically, alumni still engaging in strenuous activities plus 1,000+ additional Kcal/week in stair climbing, walking, and other light activities had less than half (42%) of the CHD incidence of their nonathletic, more sedentary classmates.

To study the influence of physical activity and such other characteristics as cigarette smoking, body mass index, hypertension, and history of parental CHD, breakpoints were used to establish three-level categories to detect any gradient effect on CHD risk. Interrelationships of paired characteristics (e.g., physical activity and smoking) at three levels each were then studied by cross-tabulation into nine resulting categories, for which CHD incidence rates were computed by the indirect method, using as standard the total 117,680 man-years observation.

Figure 1 presents a stereogram where each bar corresponds to an incidence rate of CHD for one of nine categories defined by cross-tabulation of Harvard student sports play and alumnus physical activity index. Relative risks are established by assigning RR = 1.00 to the incidence rate (85

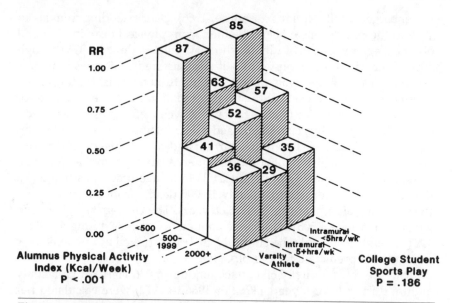

Figure 1 Incidence rates and relative risks (RR) of CHD (nonfatal or fatal) per 10,000 man-years of observation, 1962-72, by alumnus physical activity index and college student sports play. To compute *p* value trends (one-tail) for one characteristic, rates were adjusted for differences in age and the paired characteristic.

per 10,000 man-years) of the back corner bar. (Other stereograms are arranged similarly.) Student athletes who discontinued their energetic activity developed as much CHD risk as alumni who had never been athletes. Student sports alone did not predict lower CHD risk later in life, but nonathletic students acquired low CHD risk if they became fully active (physical activity index 2,000+ Kcal/week) as alumni. These trends reveal that adequate physical exercise in adult life is independent of hereditary or youthful fitness in predicting low CHD risk.

Figure 2 shows that at each level of cigarette smoking, there is a decline in CHD risk as exercise increases, and when the data are adjusted for the influence of smoking, exercise continues to be inversely related to CHD risk. Cigarette habit is directly related to CHD risk when exercise is held constant. The most active nonsmokers have only 29% the CHD risk of sedentary heavy smokers, and the most physically active heavy smokers, 56%.

Figure 3 shows that CHD risk is inversely related to exercise when weight-for-height is held constant. When exercise level is held constant, CHD risk also is significantly associated with weight, but less strongly than with physical activity index. The most active lean alumni, i.e., those no more than 10% above "ideal" weight (physical activity index 2,000+ Kcal/week and body mass index <34 units), have only 35% the CHD risk

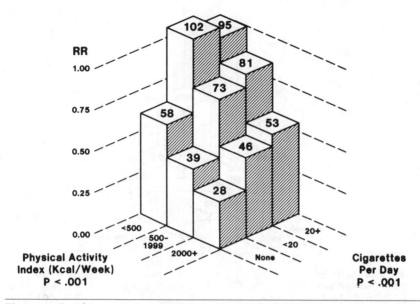

Figure 2 Incidence rates and relative risks (RR) of CHD (nonfatal or fatal) per 10,000 man-years of observation, 1962-72, by alumnus physical activity index and cigarette smoking habit. To compute *p* value trends (one-tail) for one characteristic, rates were adjusted for differences in age and the paired characteristic.

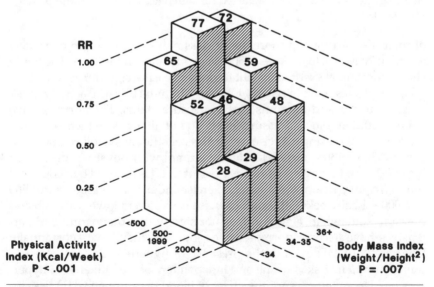

Figure 3 Incidence rates and relative risks (RR) of CHD (nonfatal or fatal) per 10,000 man-years of observation, 1962-72, by alumnus physical activity index and body mass index (1000 × weight in pounds/height in inches squared). To compute *p* value trends (one-tail) for one characteristic, rates were adjusted for differences in age and the paired characteristic.

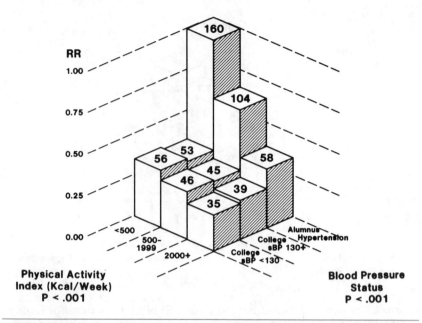

Figure 4 Incidence rates and relative risks (RR) of CHD (nonfatal or fatal) per 10,000 man-years of observation, 1962-72, by alumnus physical activity index and blood pressure status. To compute p value trends (one-tail) for one characteristic, rates were adjusted for differences in age and the paired characteristic.

of their least active and more obese classmates 20% or more over ideal weight (physical activity index <500 and body mass index 36+). The figure shows substantial exercise benefit for men in each weight-for-height class.

Figure 4 gives relative risks of CHD by alumnus physical activity index versus student and alumnus blood pressure status. For normotensive alumni, student blood pressure levels do not alter risk, which is 10-20% lower with increasing exercise, regardless of student systolic blood pressure (<130 or 130+ mmHg). Among alumni with physician-diagnosed hypertension, however, the relative risk of CHD is reduced by about two-thirds (relative risk of 0.36) when exercise index is increased from <500 to 2,000+ Kcal/week. Although exercise is known to lower casual blood pressure somewhat, Figure 4 does not signify that the vigorous hypertensives have become normotensives, but that they have substantially lower risk of CHD even in the presence of hypertension. The effect of exercise on CHD risk is strong and independent of the influence of hypertension. The reverse trend, the effect of blood pressure on CHD risk, independent of the effect of exercise, is equally strong.

Figure 5 depicts relationships of alumnus exercise level and history of parental CHD to alumnus CHD risk. To the extent that the stereogram reflects a familial or hereditary tendency toward development of CHD,

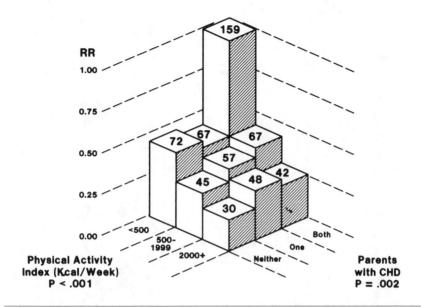

Figure 5 Incidence rates and relative risks (RR) of CHD (nonfatal or fatal) per 10,000 man-years of observation, 1962-72, by alumnus physical activity index and parental history of CHD. To compute p value trends (one-tail) for one characteristic, rates were adjusted for differences in age and the paired characteristic.

the relative risk implied by that tendency is reduced to about one-quarter (relative risk of 0.26) among alumni whose exercise index is 2,000+ Kcal/week, even if they have a double parental history of CHD. In all categories here, as in the other stereograms, there is a consistent lowering of relative risk of CHD as alumnus exercise increases from <500 to 2,000+ Kcal/week. The trend of lower CHD risk with increasing exercise is substantial, and the influence of parental CHD status on the trend of alumnus CHD risk also is strong.

Table 2 presents relative and attributable risks of first attack of CHD (nonfatal or fatal) by presence versus absence of each of five adverse characteristics, adjusted for differences in age, follow-up interval, and each of the other characteristics listed. Thus, in this multivariate model, alumni who expended <2,000 Kcal/week in walking, stair climbing, and sports play were at 49% excess risk (relative risk 1.49) of first CHD attack over men more active (relative risk 1.00). Similarly, cigarette smokers were at 30% higher risk than nonsmokers; men one-fifth or more over ideal weight-for-height (body mass index 36+) were at 32% higher risk than men less ponderous; hypertensives had 134% higher risk than normotensives; and alumni with history of parental CHD were at 28% excess risk over their classmates without such history. Each of these adverse characteristics contributes independently to CHD risk.

Table 2 Relative and Attributable Risks of First Attack of Coronary Heart Disease (CHD) (Nonfatal or Fatal) Among 16,936 Harvard Alumni, 1962-72, by Selected Adverse Characteristics

Alumnus Characteristic	Prevalence, Man-Years Observation, %	Relative Risk (1 SE) of CHD	p	Clinical Attributable Risk, %	Community Attributable Risk, %
Sedentary lifestyle[a]	61	1.49 (0.18)	< .001	33	23
Cigarette smoking[b]	52	1.30 (0.14)	.008	23	13
Overweight-for-height[c]	38	1.32 (0.14)	.005	24	11
Hypertension[d]	9	2.34 (0.31)	< .001	57	10
History of parental CHD[e]	39	1.28 (0.14)	.012	22	10

Note. Adjusted for differences in age, follow-up interval, and each of the other characteristics listed. From "A Natural History of Athleticism and Cardiovascular Health" by R.S. Paffenbarger, Jr., R.T. Hyde, A.L. Wing, and C.H. Steinmetz, 1984, *Journal of the American Medical Association,* **252**(4), p. 494. Copyright 1984, American Medical Association.

[a]Energy expenditure of < 2,000 kilocalories per week in walking, stair climbing, and sports play. [b]Any amount. [c]20% or more over ideal weight-for-height (1959 Metropolitan Life Insurance Company standards), i.e., BMI 36+. [d]Physician-diagnosed. [e]Either or both parents.

In a clinical sense, the sedentary lifestyle among less active men could account for 33% of their CHD risk; the cigarette habit, for 23% of smokers' risk; inadequate weight control, for 24% of risk among the hefty; hypertension, for 57% of hypertensives' risk; and an adverse parental history could account for 22% of the CHD risk among men reporting one or both parents to have developed clinically recognized CHD.

The impact of these adverse characteristics in the population at large is expressed as community-attributable risks percentage. The table shows that the incidence rates of first CHD attack among the Harvard alumni would have been reduced by 23% if all men had maintained a physically active lifestyle (physical activity index 2,000+ Kcal/week); by 13% if none had smoked cigarettes; 11% if all had avoided excessive overweight (body mass index 36+); 10% if none had been hypertensive; and 10% if none had had family background favoring CHD. The Harvard alumni together would have lowered their CHD risk (incidence rate) by nearly two thirds if none of the tabulated adverse characteristics had been present in their lives.

Attributable risk estimates require several assumptions: that the association between the adverse trait and CHD risk is causal and dose-dependent, that any other characteristics influencing risk are equally distributed among the levels of the traits being studied, and that those being assessed are amenable to behavioral management.

Recent Supporting Studies

W.B. Kannel and P. Sorlie (1979) followed 1,909 men and 2,311 women of Framingham, Massachusetts, who originally were without CHD. Mortality over 14 years of follow-up, especially CHD mortality, was inversely related to exercise level in the men but not the women. This largely sedentary population was administered a simplified interview questionnaire that evaluated physical activity level by hours of rest and occupational and non-occupational pursuits rated as sedentary, light, moderate, or heavy on the basis of estimated oxygen consumption. The investigators could not demonstrate physical inactivity to be a powerful characteristic favoring CHD, although some important unexplained influence was apparent. They concluded that such urban populations should engage in more vigorous exercise, especially as sedentariness and CHD risk tended to increase with age. T.R. Dawber (1980) analyzed some of the same data using somewhat different methods and a longer follow-up, reaching similar conclusions.

P. Leren et al. reported in 1975 on CHD risk among all Oslo men aged 40-49 and a 7% random sample of men aged 20-39. Men rated highly active at work were at greater risk than men with sedentary jobs but highly active in their leisure time. This may represent a blue-collar/white-collar selectivity involving other lifestyle differences. Also, it may reflect possible advantages of leisure-time exercise programmed and designed to suit the individual. This concept is worth consideration as leisure-time exercise gains prominence in the lifestyles of people everywhere.

Magnus, Matroos, and Strackee (1979) conducted a case-control study of first CHD attack, by levels of leisure-time walking, cycling, and gardening, in four residential areas in central Holland, 1970-74. Patients (or their nearest surving kin) were interviewed, as were 875 randomly chosen CHD-free control subjects living in Zeist in 1972. Exercise levels were defined as *habitual* (more than 8 months per year), *seasonal* (4-8 months), or *occasional* (less than 4 months), and by participation in hours per week. Habitual-level activities and CHD events were significantly inverse in relationship. In contrast, seasonal or occasional activities did not predict lower CHD risk. The effect from habitual-level activities was not dose-dependent on hours per week of walking, cycling, and gardening, nor did vigorous participation show any added influence. The case-fatality ratio (death within 4 weeks of CHD onset) was highest in the least active subjects, i.e., the occasional exercisers. The findings suggest that the CHD risk is reduced by year-round (habitual) leisure-time exercise, but the benefit may disappear if activity becomes intermittent.

In extending from the Seven Countries study (Keys, 1980), M. Karvonen (1982) followed two Finnish cohorts for a total of 15 years for CHD mortality and total mortality, assessing exercise levels by a detailed study of physical activity through an extensive, prestructured interview. Cross-sectional study strongly related sedentary habits to atherosclerotic trends (CHD, stroke, and claudication) in men aged 50-69. In a 5-year follow-up of 1,310 men, both CHD mortality and total mortality were inversely associated with habitual exercise. However, most CHD decedents had CHD at the outset of observations. In a subset initially free of CHD, mortality from this cause was unrelated to exercise, but combined incidence rates of myocardial infarction and CHD death declined somewhat from the least to most active study groups.

Salonen, Puska, and Tuomilehto (1982), in a 7-year longitudinal study of physical exercise and fatal and nonfatal cardiovascular disease and stroke among 7,666 Finnish men and women aged 30-59, found that low physical activity at work increased acute myocardial infarction, cerebral stroke, and mortality from any disease. The analysis adjusted for differences in age, serum total cholesterol, diastolic blood pressure, height, weight, and smoking. Low physical activity at work led to acute myocardial infarction relative risks of 1.5 in men and 2.4 in women, in contrast to workers most energetic on the job. Low activity in leisure time significantly increased risk of death in the first two years of follow-up, but not of acute myocardial infarction or stroke. Exercise level was based on response to one multiple-choice question. Risks of cardiovascular disease were significantly increased in individuals with low energy output both at work and at leisure. The findings for leisure-time exercise were less consistent than for occupational activity level, perhaps because they were confounded by smoking or other leisure-time activities. However, since physical activity may enhance favorable serum lipids and HDL-cholesterol, the analysis probably should not have adjusted for them, as adjusting for cholesterol levels could also be controlling for exercise and could mask measurements instead of sharpening them.

Garcia-Palmieri, Costas, Cruz-Vidal, Sorlie, and Havlik (1982) reported an 8.5 year follow-up study of 2,585 rural and 6,208 urban Puerto Rico men aged 45-65. They found an inverse association between exercise and risk of CHD (here not including angina pectoris), as assessed by a Framingham physical activity index. A metabolic equivalence analysis for activity likewise showed that men with vigorous exercise habits had 50% less CHD than sedentary men. Findings were similar to the results already mentioned for British civil servants, San Francisco longshoremen, and U.S. college alumni. The influences of physical activity were independent of other characteristics known to affect CHD risk—cigarette smoking, obesity, hypertension, faster heart rate, and higher levels of serum cholesterol. Omitting the first 2.5 years of follow-up to avoid premonitory selection left little difference in results. At the highest activity level, non-smokers were still at reduced CHD risk, but smokers had an increased risk. This prospective epidemiologic study was conducted in a rural area with CHD rate only about half that of the mainland, and the investigator concluded, ''The benefits from the higher activity levels in Puerto Rico probably reflect a lifetime pattern of steady activity rather than a recent increase in exercise.''

Pomrehn, Wallace, and Burmeister (1982) studied 62,000 deaths among Iowa men aged 20-64, finding that physically active farmers had 10% lower CHD mortality rates than non-farmers. The farmers had higher caloric intake and slightly higher cholesterol levels and body-mass index, but were less obese by skinfold test, and their frequencies of cigarette use and alcohol consumption were less than half of non-farmers'. The farmers were physically active twice as often, had higher HDL-cholesterol levels, and were more fit by treadmill test than non-farmers. The lower CHD mortality risk for farmers was credited to their healthier lifestyle (including less smoking). They consumed more calories because they did more physical work and needed the additional food, but their energy output was sufficient to avoid obesity and elevated serum LDL-cholesterol. It shows further that a diet coupled with a vigorous exercise program is preferable to reduction of caloric intake without adequate exercise (Wood, 1983).

Studies have found that risk of primary cardiac arrest was less than half as great in persons who had high-intensity leisure-time activity demanding at least 60% of maximum oxygen uptake, compared with persons without such exercise (Siscovick, Weiss, Fletcher, & Lasky, 1984; Siscovick, Weiss, Fletcher, Schoenback, & Wagner, 1984; Siscovick, Weiss, Hallstrom, Inui, & Peterson, 1982). The findings held in the presence or absence of hypertension, obesity, and adverse parental history of CHD. Risk of primary cardiac arrest was heightened during exercise, but much more among men only occasionally active than among those more frequently active. The analysis included only subjects who had no record of prior morbidity and had been able to be active. Personal and exercise data were gathered by telephone interviews with spouses of primary cardiac arrest decedents and matched controls; exercise levels were established much as in the U.S. college alumni study. Yet, efforts to avoid possible selection or bias reduced the roster of decedents from 1,250 to 163 (about 13%). Also, the testimony of bereaved spouses might be of questionable validity, but no special bias was found.

Peters, Cady, Bischoff, Berstein, and Pike (1983) studied 2,779 healthy public safety officers of Los Angeles County for level of physical fitness, as measured by bicycle ergometer tests, and risk of first symptomatic myocardial infarction in 13,317 man-years of follow-up. Men aged 35-54 were rated into categories below or above median values of fitness, blood pressure, total serum cholesterol, body weight, body-mass index, lean body mass, and usual activity level. Cigarette smoking and family history of heart disease were recorded as present or absent. Within an average follow-up of 5 years, 36 men had myocardial infarctions (5 fatal). The subjects below median fitness were at more than double the risk of CHD than men more fit, with adjustment for other influences. Men at highest risk were chiefly smokers or above median in cholesterol and blood pressure levels. Those less fit with any two or all three of these traits had at least six times greater risk of myocardial infarction than men more fit with the same characteristics.

In laboratory studies Kramsch, Aspen, Abramowitz, Kreimendahl, and Hood (1981) found that adequate conditioning exercise could retard coronary and other large-vessel atherosclerosis in monkeys. Treadmill-exercised and sedentary adult male *Macaca fascicularis* monkeys were compared for ischemic electrocardiographic changes, angiographic signs of coronary artery narrowing, and for gross and microscopic pathological findings. The exercised monkeys had lowered heart rates at rest and after exercise, increased heart size, a loss and regain of body weight (probably exchanging body fat for body lean), small increases in HDL-cholesterol and large decreases in total LDL- and VLDL-triglycerides, and little change in blood pressure levels. Moderate exercise also reduced coronary surface involvement and lesion size (intimal thickening), suppressed collagen accumulation, and widened lumina, in contrast to findings in sedentary animals. Retarded lesion growth in exercised monkeys was accompanied by inhibited atherosclerotic change in the aorta and other arteries. These experimental studies strongly support the findings from epidemiologic observations reported above.

Summary

Epidemiologic studies have clearly demonstrated a strong inverse relationship between physical activity and CHD risk. British studies of transport workers and civil servants, along with American studies of dock workers and college men, have provided convincing evidence that contemporary physical activity is accompanied by lower risk of both fatal and nonfatal CHD. The relationship is largely separate from such high-risk influences as cigarette smoking, hypertension, obesity, and an adverse family history of CHD. Observations on a population of college men have shown inverse relationships between exercise level and mortality from all causes, a broad array of cardiovascular conditions, and respiratory diseases; however, the relationship to cancer mortality or unnatural causes of death is less strong. The questions we need to address now are not whether exercise is a true benefit for cardiovascular and metabolic fitness, but what kind of exercise is needed and how much for optimal health. Epidemiology will continue to play a role in etiologically oriented investigations of physical activity, other personal characteristics, and chronic disease risk. In future years it also will be useful in evaluating the long-term effects of behavioral management and intervention programs only now being implemented on community-wide bases.

References

Brand, R.J., Paffenbarger, R.S., Jr., Sholtz, R.I., & Kampert, J.B. (1979). Work activity and fatal heart attack studied by multiple logistic risk analysis. *American Journal of Epidemiology*, **110**, 52-62.

Brunner, D., Manelis, G., Modan, M., & Levin, S. (1974). Physical activity at work and the incidence of myocardial infarction, angina pectoris, and death due to ischemic heart disease: An epidemiological study in Israeli collective settlements (kibbutzim). *Journal of Chronic Diseases*, **27**, 217-233.

Cassel, J., Heyden, S., Bartel, A.C., Kaplan, B.H., Tyroler, H.A., Cornoni, J.C., & Hames, C.G. (1971). Occupation and physical activity and coronary heart disease. *Archives of Internal Medicine*, **128**, 920-928.

Chapman, J.M., & Massey, F.J. (1964). The interrelationship of serum cholesterol, hypertension, body weight, and risk of coronary heart disease: Results of the first ten years follow-up in the Los Angeles heart study. *Journal of Chronic Diseases*, **17**, 933-947.

Chave, S.P.W., Morris, J.N., Moss, S., & Semmence, A.M. (1978). Vigorous exercise in leisure time and the death rate: A study of male civil servants. *Journal of Epidemiology and Community Health*, **32**, 239-243.

Dawber, T.R. (1980). The Framingham study. In *The epidemiology of atherosclerotic disease* (pp. 151-171). Cambridge, MA: Harvard University Press.

Epstein, L., Miller, G.J., Stitt, F.W., & Morris, J.N. (1976). Vigorous exercise in leisure time, coronary risk factors, and resting electrocardiogram in middle-aged civil servants. *British Heart Journal*, **38**, 403-409.

Garcia-Palmieri, M.R., Costas, R., Jr., Cruz-Vidal, M., Sorlie, P.D., & Havlik, R.S. (1982). Increased physical activity: A protective factor against heart attacks in Puerto Rico. *American Journal of Cardiology*, **50**, 749-755.

Kahn, H.A. (1963). The relationship of reported coronary heart disease mortality to physical activity of work. *American Journal of Public Health*, **53**, 1058-1067.

Kannel, W.B., & Sorlie, P. (1979). Some health benefits of physical activity: The Framingham study. *Archives of Internal Medicine*, **139**, 857-861.

Karvonen, M.J. (1981). Occupation, daily activities, and leisure as sources of fitness and health. *Hermes (Leuven)*, **15**, 303-323.

Karvonen, M.J. (1982). Physical activity in work and leisure time in relation to cardiovascular diseases. *Annals of Clinical Research*, **14**(Suppl. 34), 118-123.

Keys, A. (1980) *Seven countries: A multivariate analysis of death and coronary heart disease*. Cambridge, MA: Harvard University Press.

Kramsch, D.M., Aspen, A.J., Abramowitz, B.M., Kreimendahl, T., & Hood, W.B., Jr. (1981). Reduction of coronary atherosclerosis by moderate conditioning exercise in monkeys on an atherogenic diet. *New England Journal of Medicine*, **305**, 1483-1489.

Leren, P., Askevold, E.M., Foss, O.P., Froili, A., Grymyr, D., Helgeland, A., Hjermann, I., Holme, I., Lund-Larsen, P.G., & Norum, K.R. (1975). The Oslo study: Cardiovascular disease in middle-aged and young Oslo men. *Acta Medica Scandinavica*, (Suppl. 588), 1-38.

Magnus, K., Matroos, A., & Strackee, J. (1979). Walking, cycling, or gardening with or without seasonal interruption in relation to acute coronary events. *American Journal of Epidemiology*, **110**, 724-733.

Menotti, A., & Puddu, V. (1976). Death rates among the Italian railroad employees, with special reference to coronary heart disease and physical activity at work. *Environmental Research*, **11**, 331-342.

Morris, J.N. (1975). *Uses of epidemiology* (3rd ed.). New York: Churchill Livingstone.

Morris, J.N., Chave, S.P.W., Adam, C., Sirey, C., Epstein, L., & Sheehan, D.J. (1973). Vigorous exercise in leisure-time and the incidence of coronary heart-disease. *Lancet*, **1**, 333-339.

Morris, J.N., Everitt, M.G., Pollard, R., Chave, S.P.W., & Semmence, A.M. (1980). Vigorous exercise in leisure-time: Protection against coronary heart-disease. *Lancet*, **2**, 1207-1210.

Morris, J.N., Heady, J.A., Raffle, P.A.B., Roberts, C.G., & Parks, J.W. (1953). Coronary heart disease and physical activity of work. *Lancet*, **2**, 1053-1057, 1111-1120.

Morris, J.N., Kagan, A., Pattison, D.C., Gardner, M., & Raffle, P.A.B. (1966). Incidence and prediction of ischaemic heart disease in London busmen. *Lancet*, **2**, 552-559.

Paffenbarger, R.S., Jr. (1977). Physical activity and fatal heart attack: Protection or selection. In E.A. Amsterdam, J.H. Wilmore, & A.N. DeMaria (Eds.), *Exercise in cardiovascular health and disease* (pp. 35-49). New York: Yorke Medical Books.

Paffenbarger, R.S., Jr., Brand, R.J., Sholtz, R.I., & Jung, D.L. (1978). Energy expenditure, cigarette smoking, and blood pressure level as related to death from specific diseases. *American Journal of Epidemiology*, **108**, 12-18.

Paffenbarger, R.S., Jr., & Hale, W.E. (1975). Work activity and coronary heart mortality. *New England Journal of Medicine*, **292**, 545-550.

Paffenbarger, R.S., Jr., Hale, W.E., Brand, R.J., & Hyde, R.T. (1977). Work-energy level, personal characteristics, and fatal heart attack: A birth-cohort effect. *American Journal of Epidemiology*, **105**, 200-213.

Paffenbarger, R.S., Jr., Hyde, R.T., Wing, A.L., & Steinmetz, C.H. (1984). A natural history of athleticism and cardiovascular health. *Journal of the American Medical Association*, **252**, 491-495.

Paffenbarger, R.S., Jr., Laughlin, M.E., Gima, A.S., & Black, R.A. (1970). Work activity of longshoremen as related to death from coronary heart disease and stroke. *New England Journal of Medicine*, **282**, 1109-1114.

Paffenbarger, R.S., Jr., Notkin, J., Krueger, D.E., Wolf, P.A., Thorne, M.C., LeBauer, E.J., & Williams, J.L. (1966). Chronic disease in former college students: II. Methods of study and observations on mortality from coronary heart disease. *American Journal of Public Health*, **56**, 962-971.

Paffenbarger, R.S., Jr., & Wing, A.L. (1969). Chronic disease in former college students: X. The effects of single and multiple characteristics on risk of fatal coronary heart disease. *American Journal of Epidemiology*, **90**, 527-535.

Paffenbarger, R.S., Jr., Wing, A.L., & Hyde, R.T. (1978). Chronic disease in former college students: XVI. Physical activity as an index of heart attack risk in college alumni. *American Journal of Epidemiology*, **108**, 161-175.

Paffenbarger, R.S., Jr., Wolf, P.A., Notkin, J., & Thorne, M.C. (1966). Chronic disease in former college students: I. Early precursors of fatal coronary heart disease. *American Journal of Epidemiology*, **83**, 314-328.

Paul, O., Lepper, M.H., Phelan, W.H., Dupertuis, G.W., MacMillan, A., McKean, H., & Park, H. (1963). A longitudinal study of coronary heart disease. *Circulation*, **28**, 20-31.

Peters, R.S., Cady, L.D., Jr., Bischoff, D.P., Bernstein, L., & Pike, M.C. (1983). Physical fitness and subsequent myocardial infarction in healthy workers. *Journal of the American Medical Association*, **249**, 3052-3056.

Pomrehn, P.R., Wallace, R.B., & Burmeister, L.F. (1982). Ischemic heart disease mortality in Iowa farmers: The influence of lifestyle. *Journal of the American Medical Association*, **248**, 1073-1076.

Ramazzini, B. (1964). *Diseases of workers* (W.C. Wright, Trans.). New York: Hafner. (Original work published 1700)

Salonen, J.T., Puska, P., & Tuomilehto, J. (1982). Physical activity and risk of myocardial infarction, cerebral stroke, and death: A longitudinal study in eastern Finland. *American Journal of Epidemiology*, **115**, 526-537.

Siscovick, D.S., Weiss, N.S., Fletcher, R.H., & Lasky, T. (1984). The incidence of primary cardiac arrest during vigorous exercise. *New England Journal of Medicine*, **311**, 874-877.

Siscovick, D.S., Weiss, N.S., Fletcher, R.H., Schoenbach, V.J., & Wagner, E.H. (1984). Habitual vigorous exercise and primary cardiac arrest: Effect of other risk factors on the relationship. *Journal of Chronic Diseases*, **37**, 625-631.

Siscovick, D.S., Weiss, N.S., Hallstrom, A.P., Inui, T.S., & Peterson, D.R. (1982). Physical activity and primary cardiac arrest. *Journal of the American Medical Association*, **248**, 3113-3117.

Stamler, J., Lindberg, H.A., Berkson, H.A., Shaffer, A., Miller, W., & Poindexter, A. (1960). Prevalence and incidence of coronary heart disease in strata of the labor force of a Chicago industrial corporation. *Journal of Chronic Diseases*, **11**, 405-420.

Taylor, H.L., Klepetar, E., Keys, A., Parlin, M.S., Blackburn, H., & Puchner, T. (1962). Death rates among physically active and sedentary employees of the railroad industry. *American Journal of Public Health*, **52**, 1697-1707.

Wood, P.D. (1983). *California diet and exercise program*. Mountain View, CA: Anderson World.

Wood, P.D., Haskell, W.L., Blair, S.N., Williams, P.T., Krauss, R.M., Lindgren, F.T., Albers, J.J., Ho, P.H., & Farquhar, J.W. (1983). Increased exercise level and plasma lipoprotein concentrations: A one-year, randomized, controlled study in sedentary, middle-aged men. *Metabolism*, **32**, 31-39.

Zukel, W.J., Lewis, R.H., Enterline, P.E., Painter, R.C., Ralston, L.S., Fawcett, R.M., Meredith, A.P., & Peterson, B. (1959). A short-term community study of the epidemiology of coronary heart disease: A preliminary report on the North Dakota study. *American Journal of Public Health*, **49**, 1630-1639.

This work was supported by the E.I. du Pont de Nemours Company; the G. Unger Vetlesen Foundation; the Sun Company, Inc.; the Union Carbide Corporation; the Exxon Corporation; the Mobil Foundation; the Marathon Oil Foundation, Inc.; the Phillips Petroleum Foundation, Inc.; and Research Grant No. HL 06859 from the National Heart, Lung, and Blood Institute.

Chapter 2

Early Intervention/ Prevention in Childhood

Debra Dodson Drake
Charles T. Kuntzleman

The major killer and crippler of North Americans is heart disease (coronary artery disease) (Public Health Service, 1965). It reduces longevity and quality of life. It frequently strikes during a person's most productive years and causes premature death or significantly reduces the survivor's productivity.

Coronary Artery Disease Risk Factors Appear in Childhood

Most people picture coronary artery disease as an illness that occurs in old age. As the following, previously reported facts show, the seeds for this disease are planted in childhood:

- By age 3 nearly all U.S. children have some fat deposits on the inner surface of the aorta, the body's largest artery. These deposits increase rapidly after age 8, and by age 15 affect an average of 15% of the aortic surface (McGill, 1980).
- In elementary schools, up to 24% of children have elevated cholesterol levels, and 15% have abnormal triglyceride levels (Lauer et al., 1975).
- Twenty percent of children 6 to 9 years of age have excess body fat (Gilliam et al., 1977; Lauer et al., 1975).
- One to 4 1/2% of the children between the ages of 3 and 18 have elevated blood pressure (Lauer et al., 1975, Londe et al., 1971).
- Sixty-two percent of children have at least one heart disease risk factor, and 36% have two or more (Gilliam et al., 1977).

- Children in the sixth, seventh, and eighth grades have a deficiency in cardiovascular health knowledge. In fact, as they get older, the deficiency becomes greater relative to their knowledge in other subject areas (White et al., 1977).
- A review of health curricula in the secondary schools of a major U.S. city revealed that only 10-15% of the health coursework was devoted to cardiovascular disease and cancer (Mroczek, 1976)—diseases that cause over 70% of all deaths. Tragically, many elementary and secondary schools do not provide any health education at all.
- Reports in the popular press point out that the fitness levels of U.S. school children are declining, schools are employing cost-cutting measures which reduce time spent on physical education, children are eating more foods low in nutrients and high in sugar, and almost one-half of elementary school children have tried smoking (Kuntzleman, 1977).

Lifetime Exercise and Dietary Habits Begin Early

Patterns of activity, eating, and outlook are established early in life. Therefore, programs should aim for control of cardiovascular risk factors early in life. The heart attack of middle age has its root in childhood. Because of the early onset of cardiovascular disease, health programs that stress behavior change should focus on children as well as adults.

Educators, however, question whether aggressive daily health promotion programs and behavior change strategies would be beneficial. They note that 30 minutes a day is only one percent of a year, hardly enough time to counter the negative health attitudes and concepts which permeate a child's environment. Furthermore, recent studies have been unable to show positive results from efforts to modify a child's risk for cardiovascular disease. Many factors have affected the results: Most of the studies were descriptive in nature, dealt with one aspect or risk, did not incorporate a control group, and did not provide a large enough number of subjects. Nevertheless, these studies have prompted the initiation of other additional research into the effects of early intervention programs.

The Feelin' Good Youth Fitness Report

A grant from the W.K. Kellogg Foundation of Battle Creek, Michigan, allowed researchers from Fitness Finders, Inc., Spring Arbor College, and the University of Michigan to evaluate (a) selected cardiovascular health factors and health habits in children 7-12 years of age, (b) the effects of the Feelin' Good program on the cardiovascular health and health habits of these children, and (c) the effects of physical fitness and body fat on selected cardiovascular risk factors and self-esteem.

The study lasted three years (1980-83) and probed the physiological characteristics of 7-, 10-, and 12-year-old boys and girls in Jackson County, Michigan, a blue-collar community. Each year 120 children (totaling 360 experimental subjects) were involved in the testing and the Feelin' Good program. From a neighboring county, another 30 children each year (for a three-year total of 90) acted as the control group. The children's cardiovascular risk factors, physical fitness levels, body weight and fat, health knowledge and health attitudes (including self-esteem, physical activity, and eating patterns) were examined.

For detailed analysis on all variables, refer to the *Technical Report of the Feelin' Good Youth Fitness Report*. A 35-page summary report and a 215-page technical report are available for purchase from Fitness Finders, Inc., 133 Teft Road, Spring Arbor, MI 49283.

Health and Fitness Status of the Children

The pretest data provided a description and evaluation of the differences and similarities between the Jackson County children and current national averages.

Physiological Data and Eating Patterns

The children were very close to the national averages in measurements of height and weight (Tables 1 and 2). Body fat levels were 2-5% above average. Blood lipids and resting blood pressures were similar to the average (Table 3). The physical fitness scores, as measured by the mile run, were similar to, or slightly above, the average (Table 4).

The children's diets were high in simple carbohydrates, total and saturated fat, protein and sodium, but low in iron, calcium and fiber (Table 5). The children ate far more poorly than recommended in the government's U.S. Dietary Guidelines for optimal health.

Physical Activity Data

In years 1 and 2 the children wore heart-rate-recording devices (Holter monitors) to determine their levels of physical activity. Although heart rates may increase for reasons other than exercise (e.g., stress, fear, or sickness), it was felt that recording heart rates in this manner provided a satisfactory method of estimating the children's physical activity patterns.

Table 1 Body Measurement Means of Feelin' Good® Boys by Age

Variables	7-Year-Olds	U.S. Average[a]	10-Year-Olds	U.S. Average	12-Year-Olds	U.S. Average
Age (yrs)	7.3	7.0	10.3	10.0	12.3	12.0
Height	4' 2.1"	4' 0"	4' 8.5"	4' 6.1"	5' 0.7"	4' 11.1"
Weight (lbs)	58.4	50.7	78.9	70.6	101.5	88.2
Skinfolds total (mm)	30.8*	—[b]	37.4	—	55.0	—
% Body fat	17.5	14	20.5	16	22.5	17.5
Chest (in)	24.1	—	27.0	—	29.9	—
Abdomen (in)	22.3	—	24.8	—	27.4	—

[a]U.S. averages are based on Parizkova (1961) and Vital Statistics Report (1976).
[b]Dash means "not available."

Table 2 Body Measurement Means of Feelin' Good® Girls by Age

Variables	7-Year-Olds	U.S. Average[a]	10-Year-Olds	U.S. Average	12-Year-Olds	U.S. Average
Age (yrs)	7.2	7.0	10.2	10.0	12.2	12.0
Height	4' 1.4"	3' 9.4"	4' 8.7"	4' 6.3"	5' 1.1"	4' 11.8"
Weight (lbs)	56.3	49.6	80.5	71.6	98.5	92.6
Skinfolds total (mm)	37.3*	—[b]	49.6	—	51.0	—
% Body fat	21.5	19	24.0	20.5	24	21.5
Chest (in)	23.9	—	27.1	—	30.4	—
Abdomen (in)	22.1	—	24.0	—	25.8	—

[a]U.S. averages are based on Parizkova (1961) and Vital Statistics Report (1976).

[b]Dash means "not available."

Table 3   Blood Lipids and Blood Pressures of Feelin' Good® Children by Age

Variables	7-Year-Olds	10-Year-Olds	12-Year-Olds
Blood Lipids			
Cholesterol	168 (162)	173 (159)	166 (159)
HDL	51 (54)	51 (54)	49 (54)
Triglycerides	72 (58)	69 (70)	79 (70)
Blood Pressures			
Resting systolic	89 (96)	97 (97)	100 (101)
Resting diastolic	59 (58)	62 (62)	66 (62)

ªNumbers in parentheses are U.S. averages based on Lipid Research Clinics (1980).

Table 4   Physical Fitness Scores of Feelin' Good® Children by Age

Variables	7-Year-Olds	10-Year-Olds	12-Year-Olds
Sit and reach (in)	11.3 (10.2)ª	10.5 (10.6)	11.3 (11.0)
Sit-ups (no./min)	27 (26)	37 (33)	39 (38)
Grip strength (lbs)	25 (23)	38 (34)	49 (45)
Mile run (min:sec)	10:09 (11:57)	8:55 (10:12)	8:54 (9:04)

ªNumbers in parentheses are U.S. averages based on American Alliance for Health, Physical Education, Recreation, and Dance (1980).

For this study the researchers used a minimal figure of 75% of maximum heart rate for the children. Therefore, a heart rate of 159 beats per minute was considered the training threshold. A training zone of 160 to 190 beats per minute was thus established for the children.

The children spent only 2% of the total 12-hour period at heart rates in the training zone (Table 6). When calculated for 24 hours the children spent 96% of the time in sedentary or mild physical activities, 3% in moderate physical activities, and 1% in vigorous activities.

The Effects of the Feelin' Good Program

The Feelin' Good intervention program was implemented for 13 weeks for the 7- and 10-year-olds, and for 9 weeks for the 12-year-olds. Thirty-

Table 5   Comparison of Feelin' Good® Children's Eating Patterns With Current U.S. Eating Patterns and U.S. Dietary Guidelines

Variables	Feelin' Good® Children	U.S. Average[b]	Dietary[c] Guidelines
Total carbohydrates	48.5%	47-50%	58%
Simple	25%	26-27% (est)	10%
Complex	23%	21-23% (est)	48%
Total fat	35%	36-38%	30%
Saturated	13.5%	16%	0%
Unsaturated	16%	15-16%	10%
Polyunsaturated	6%	5-6%	10%
Protein	16%	14%	12%
Cholesterol (mg)	283	220-312	300

[a]There were virtually no differences between the boys and girls or ages, so they were combined.

[b]Data from Lipid Research Clinics (1982).

[c]Data from *Nutrition and Your Health* (1980).

minute exercise sessions four times a week were initiated. Two 30-minute classroom sessions were also held each week.

Physiological Effects

In comparing the Feelin' Good group to the control group, it was found that the Feelin' Good children had a 16% decrease in skinfold measurements (Table 7). These changes were collectively most evident among the 10- and 12-year-olds.

In looking at the children by sex and age, the Feelin' Good girls showed the greatest change. There also seemed to be a slowing of chest and waist girth increase among the 12-year-old girls.

Physical Fitness

There were significant improvements in the mile run times among the Feelin' Good children, compared to the control children (Table 7). The Feelin' Good children decreased their times an average of 61 seconds, whereas the control children decreased 22 seconds.

The Feelin' Good children consistently had better posttest mile run times than the control children. This was particularly true of the girls. At pretest,

Table 6   Comparison of Heart Rate Data Between Feelin' Good® and Control Children

Heart Rate/Min (% of 12 hrs)	Feelin' Good® Children		Control Children		Effect
	Pre	Post	Pre	Post	
Less than 100 (% of 12 hrs)	400 min 56%	362 min 50%	412 min 57%	437 min 61%	NS
100 to 129 (% of 12 hrs)	263 min 36%	284 min 40%	237 min 33%	228 min 32%	NS
130 to 159 (% of 12 hrs)	43 min 6%	52 min 7%	47 min 7%	46 min 6%	NS
More than 159 (% of 12 hrs)	14 min 2%	22 min 3%	24 min 3%	9 min 1%	NS

Table 7   Summary of Selected Effects

Variable/Group	n	Pretest	Posttest	p Value
Skinfolds total (mm)				
Feelin' Good	349	43.5	41.3	< .001
Control	85	41.9	46.6	
Mile run (min:sec)				
Feelin' Good	313	9:19	8:18	< .001
Control	85	9:27	9.05	
TOT-C (mg)				
Feelin' Good	207	169.0	165.2	< .05
Control	55	164.2	166.6	
Resting systolic blood pressure				
Feelin' Good	341	95.5	92.1	NS
Control	86	101.9	96.9	
Resting diastolic blood pressure				
Feelin' Good	341	62.3	58.8	< .001
Control	86	66.0	66.0	

the Feelin' Good girls at all age levels had poorer mile run times than the control girls, yet at posttest the Feelin' Good girls' times were substantially better than those of control girls.

Blood Lipids and Resting Blood Pressures

Total cholesterol values of the Feelin' Good children decreased significantly in comparison to the control group's slight increase (Table 7).

There were moderate but nonsignificant decreases in the resting systolic blood pressure of both the Feelin' Good and control children (Table 7). However, the diastolic blood pressure of the Feelin' Good children showed a significant 6% reduction. In fact, regardless of age or sex, the Feelin' Good children had decreases in their resting diastolic blood pressure.

Stress Test

The Feelin' Good children had a significant increase in their level of work at the completion of the stress test (Table 8). The improvement of this variable suggested a higher potential of the children to do exercise. The Feelin' Good children also did significantly more total work than the control children. There was no difference in peak heart rate or peak systolic blood pressure between the Feelin' Good children and the control group.

The Feelin' Good children, therefore, were able to do more work without appreciable increases in systolic blood pressure or peak heart rate. This is an indication that the Feelin' Good children's cardiovascular systems were more efficient than those of the control children.

Eating Patterns

No significant changes were found in total caloric intake (the Feelin' Good children ate approximately 50 fewer calories a day; the control children ate approximately 60 more calories a day). Total carbohydrate intake by the Feelin' Good group showed a moderate reduction, primarily due to a significant decrease in simple carbohydrate consumption (Table 8).

Significant differences in total fat consumption were found only among the 12-year-old Feelin' Good girls. These girls also showed significant differences in saturated, unsaturated, and polyunsaturated fat intakes. There was an appreciable but nonsignificant 3% decrease in sodium intake among the Feelin' Good children.

The eating pattern data in this investigation demonstrated that the Feelin' Good program had a small, but positive, effect on the children's eating patterns.

Table 8 Summary of Selected Effects

Variable/Group	N	Pretest	Posttest	(p Value)
Watt peak (kpm/min)				
Feelin' Good	207	101.2	108.8	< .05
Control	53	103.2	105.9	
Cum watt (kpm/min)				
Feelin' Good	207	484.5	549.4	< .001
Control	53	528.9	509.2	
Peak HR (bts/min)				
Feelin' Good	207	195.0	190.9	NS
Control	53	196.9	193.4	
Peak SBP (mmHg)				
Feelin' Good	207	142.1	149.2	NS
Control	53	142.6	148.9	
Calories				
Feelin' Good	308	1980.0	1927.9	NS
Control	73	1940.0	1999.8	
Total carbohydrates				
Feelin' Good	308	234.3	224.3	Trend (p = .07)
Control	73	220.8	233.6	
Complex carbohydrates				
Feelin' Good	308	111.7	108.9	NS
Control	73	109.7	112.9	
Simple carbohydrates				
Feelin' Good	308	122.6	115.4	< .05
Control	73	111.1	120.7	

Physical Activity Patterns

To determine how hard the children were exercising in the Feelin' Good workout and in the traditional physical education classroom, the children checked their heart rates daily by personal or teacher palpitation, and/or with Exersentry equipment. Heart rates were checked 10 and 18 minutes into activity. Personal daily reports were kept.

The data in Figure 1 show that at all ages the Feelin' Good children had significantly higher heart rates at both 10 and 18 minutes. The Feelin' Good children had heart rates which averaged 170.5 beats per minute during the peak phase of the workout. They were exercising, on the average, at 81% of their predicted maximum heart rate. The traditional physical education children had heart rates averaging 111.5 beats per minute, or 53% of their predicted maximum heart rate.

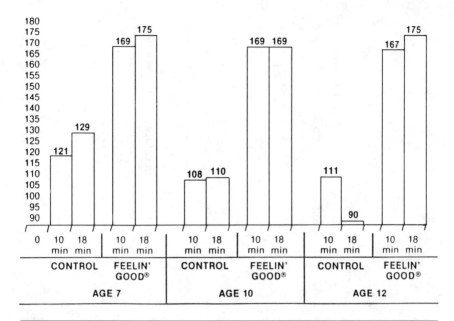

Figure 1 Comparison of Feelin' Good® and control children's heart rates at 10 and 18 minutes into the active phases of the Feelin' Good® and traditional physical education workouts.

In comparing the heart rates for an entire 12-hour period (Table 6), no significant difference was found between the Feelin' Good and control children, probably due to the small number (3) of control subjects. Nevertheless, there was a 15% reduction in the time the Feelin' Good children spent in sedentary activities and a 46% increase in the time they spent in moderate and vigorous physical activities.

Fitness Levels—Effects on Cardiovascular Risk Factors

The children's fitness levels were compared with selected physiological risk factor variables. The fitness levels were determined from the age-adjusted mile run time categories established from the American Alliance for Health, Physical Education, Recreation, and Dance (AAHPERD) percentile norms.

When the fitness levels were compared to cardiovascular risk factors, a direct inverse relationship was seen; that is, when the children's cardiovascular fitness levels went up, their cardiovascular risk factors declined (Table 9). The cardiovascular risk factors affected significantly were

Table 9 Physical Fitness Levels Versus Selected Risk Factors Feelin' Good® and Control Children Pretest Data

| Fitness Level | Risk Factor Variables | | | | | Blood Pressure | |
	Cholesterol (mg/100 ml)	HDL	HDL/TOT-C	Triglycerides (mg/100 ml)	Skinfolds (mm)	Systolic (mm Hg)	Diastolic (mm Hg)
Very poor	164	38	18	122	125	121	86
Poor	166	45	24	86	81[A]	106[a]	65[A]
Average	167	49[f]	26	77	46[A.B]	99[A.b]	65[A]
Good	170	50[f]	27[a.b.]	72[A]	36[A.B.C]	95[A.B.C]	60[A.C]
Excellent	167	50[f]	30[A.B.C]	73[A]	33[A.B.C]	92[A.B.C.d]	62[A]

Significance   Trends

a [A]Significant in comparison to Very Poor   [f] Trend in comparison to Very Poor

b [B]Significant in comparison to Poor

c [C]Significant in comparison to Average

d [D]Significant in comparison to Good

a type: < .05

A type: < .01

HDL/TOT-C, triglycerides, skinfolds, and systolic and diastolic blood pressures.

Conclusion

The children in Jackson County, Michigan, initially were representative of American children. Their body measurements, fitness scores, blood pressures and lipids, eating and physical activity patterns, and cardiovascular disease risk factors were very similar to the average.

It is our conclusion that aerobic-based programs such as Feelin' Good are effective in modifying children's cardiovascular fitness and physical activity and eating patterns, and in reducing cardiovascular disease risk factors. Consider the following:

- The stress test data in the Feelin' Good study demonstrated that the children involved in an aerobic-based exercise program improved their ability to withstand vigorous exercise. Significant improvements in total and peak work scores, without significant increases in peak heart rates and systolic blood pressures, were indicators of better exercise tolerance.
- The eating pattern data in the Feelin' Good study demonstrated that the Feelin' Good program seemed to have a small, but positive, effect on the children's eating patterns.
- The tendencies for less weight gain and girth measures, along with significant skinfold reductions, support the observation that an aerobic-based exercise program can be effective in reducing children's body fat.
- Blood cholesterol and resting diastolic blood pressure showed a significant decrease when the children were involved in an aerobic-based program of exercise.
- The Feelin' Good study showed that as fitness levels increased, cardiovascular disease risk factors decreased.

The data from the Feelin' Good study shows objectively what experts have been stating subjectively for the past few decades: Cardiovascular disease risk-reduction programs can and should be started with children.

References

American Alliance for Health, Physical Education, Recreation, and Dance. (1980). *Life time health related physical fitness test manual*. Reston, VA: Author.

Gilliam, T.B., et al. (1977). Prevalence of coronary heart disease risk factors in active children, 7 to 12 years of age. *Medicine and Science in Sports,* **9**, 21.

Kuntzleman, C.T. (1977). *Color me red!* Spring Arbor, MI: Arbor Press.

Lauer, R.M., et al. (1975). The coronary heart disease risk factors in school children: The Muscatine study. *Journal of Pediatrics,* **86**, 697.

Londe, S., et al. (1971). Hypertension in apparently normal children. *Journal of Pediatrics,* **78**, 569.

McGill, H.C., Jr. (1980). Morphologic development of the atherosclerotic plaque. In R.M. Lauer & R.B. Shekelle (Eds.), *Childhood prevention of atherosclerosis and hypertension* (pp. 41-50). New York: Raven Press.

Mroczek, W.J. (1976). High school health curriculum: A neglected medical resource. *American Heart Journal,* **92**, 271.

National Center for Health Statistics. (1976, June 22). *Vital statistics report: NCHS growth charts* (Vol. 25, No. 3). Washington, DC: Author.

National Institutes of Health. (1980). *The lipid research clinics population studies data book: Vol. 1. The prevalence study* (U.S. Dept. of Health and Human Services, Public Health Service, Publication No. 80-1527). Bethesda, MD: Author.

National Institutes of Health. (1982). *The lipid research clinics population studies data book: Vol. II. The prevalence study—nutrient intake* (U.S. Dept. of Health and Human Services, Public Health Service, Publication No. 82-2014). Bethesda, MD: Author.

Parizkova, J. (1961). Total body fat and skinfold thickness in children. *Metabolism,* **10**, 794.

U.S. Department of Agriculture, Office of Governmental and Public Affairs. (1980). *Nutrition and your health: Dietary guidelines for Americans.* Washington, DC: Author.

U.S. Department of Health, Education, and Welfare, Public Health Service. (1965). *Coronary heart disease in adults, United States 1960-62* (Data from the National Survey, Vital and Health Statistics 11, No. 10). Washington, DC: Author.

White, C.W., et al. (1977). The status of cardiovascular health knowledge among sixth, seventh, and eighth grade children. *Circulation,* **56**, 480.

Chapter 3

Motivation for a Lifetime of Involvement

Debra Dodson Drake
Charles T. Kuntzleman

Attrition is a word that makes fitness leaders cringe. We take it personally when a person drops out or simply fails to attend our exercise program regularly. We question ourselves, "What's wrong with my personality? Don't they like the program, or is it our facility? Should I play different music?" Why shouldn't we take it personally, when Webster defines attrition as "the act of wearing away by friction" (*Webster's New Universal*, 1979).

Dropouts from physical activity programs are common. Over 50% of adults who join programs leave before completion (*Sticking With Fitness*, 1982). Researchers have studied why some people start programs and stay with them but others start only to drop out. A review of current research provides some revealing information:

- Dropouts are more likely to be single than married and to be younger than older (Olson & Zanna, 1982).
- People who are overweight tend to drop out more frequently (Dishman, Ickes, & Morgan, 1980).
- Smokers report less physical activity than nonsmokers and also are more likely to drop an exercise program (Olson, 1982).
- Persons who do not receive support from their spouses are more likely to be dropouts (Wankel, 1981).
- People who are depressed or hostile are frequent dropouts (Ho et al., 1981).
- People who do not have a tendency to persevere are less likely to stay with a program of exercise (Dishman, 1980).

- Dropout rates are higher for jogging and calisthenics than other types of exercise (*Those Who Know*, 1982).
- The occurrence of injuries is one of the best predictors for dropouts (Martin & Smith, 1981).
- High intensity exercise is another good predictor for dropouts (Martin, 1981).
- Participants who do not achieve their goals in exercise programs drop out approximately twice as early as those who do (Buffone, Sachs, & Dowd, 1979).

Many exercise program directors have used such observations to evaluate participant adherence. We may have been looking at the problem from the wrong angle: Instead of looking solely at the negative aspect, attrition, we need to look at the positive, why people continue to exercise. Adherence, "the state of sticking, a steady attachment" (*Webster's New Universal*, 1979) is the aspect we need to evaluate.

- People often initiate exercise for improvement of health, but reasons for continued activity change from health to enjoyment factors (Perrin, 1979).
- A sense of personal commitment to continue is often a motivating factor for participants who stay with an exercise program (Perrin, 1979).
- Participants who have realistic goals and monitor their progress adhere better to a program of exercise (Wankel, 1979).
- Exercising with others (Franklin, 1978) and making friends in an exercise group (Wankel, 1981) encourage individuals to stay with a program.
- Input in the choice of activities prompts participants to adhere to an exercise program (Thompson & Wankel, 1980).
- Supportive and attentive exercise leaders are a must (Wankel, 1981).
- Personal feedback will prompt individuals to stay more than group feedback or no feedback (Martin, Katell, Webster, Zegman, & Blount, 1981).
- Maintaining a daily record and monitoring progress toward goals encourage continued involvement (Brownell & Stunkard, 1980).
- Rewards have a positive impact on adherence of most exercise participants (Keefe & Blumenthal, 1980).

The reasons for adult dropout and adherence give some idea of how to motivate children for lifetime involvement in physical activity. The areas of effective approach have been generalized into five categories—education, environment, self-esteem, goals and values, and enjoyment.

Education

Education should be a major component of every program of exercise. If education is not included, the program is dealing with the rehabilitative, or at most the preventive, aspect of health, not wellness. Rehabilitative and preventive programs currently have their places, but proper exercise programs should provide the participants with a sense of taking charge of their own health. Education provides the means for a participant to take this responsibility and make intelligent decisions concerning his or her behavior.

It is difficult for young people to appreciate the immediate importance of working to prevent diseases that may not manifest themselves for several decades. Most young adults and children appear to be quite healthy and energetic. However, research had documented that cardiovascular disease begins in childhood (Kuntzleman & Drake, 1984). Patterns of activity, eating, and outlook are established early in life. Current information regarding potential risk, therefore, must be made available to children. An awareness must be created. Programs must then provide children with the proper tools to manage current health situations effectively and avoid future disease.

Overweight individuals have a higher rate of attrition. Children need to be instructed early in the concepts of weight control. They need to understand why obesity is a health problem, the dangers and fallacies of fad diets, proper nutrition, and how exercise is the proper method for weight control. Children also need to know they are not expected to be perfect. They need to know it is okay to falter or fail, and that persons must deal with their own bodies and needs.

Smokers also tend to be exercise dropouts. An early educational program is needed to provide children not only with facts about smoking, but also with positive alternatives (e.g., exercise, hobbies). Hypothetical situations can produce values and thought patterns that will be effective in countering peer pressure in real-life situations.

The educational aspect should also provide students with basic knowledge of what type of exercise is best and how much is enough. *The Feelin' Good Youth Fitness Report* (Kuntzleman & Drake, 1984) established that instruction on exercise concepts is necessary. Children view their activity in perspective of how active their parents are. When children comprehend concepts of exercise and how much they need, healthy behavior patterns are established early in life. Proper education should also aid in preventing injuries and boredom, two major causes of attrition.

Education provides students with a sense of control over their present and future health. This is important. A 1983 nationwide survey taken by

Louis Harris and Association, Inc. found that those adults who felt they had control over their future health were more likely to practice preventive behavior.

Environment

The environmental aspect of motivating children includes not only the facility itself, but more importantly, support from peers, community, family, school, and the medical profession. The convenience of the facility location and class scheduling is an important factor among adults (Wankel, 1981). The facility can be made more appealing to children by allowing them to help make their playground attractive and conducive for active play.

More than just a pleasant, convenient facility is needed for lifetime involvement, though. Moral support is a necessity, whether it be from friends, spouses, exercise leaders, or even the media. Rod Dishman (1984) showed that for the adult exercise participant, the attitude of the spouse is more influential in adherence than the attitude of the participant. For children, creating a positive school or community environment provides support. Dr. Charles Kuntzleman (1984) noted, "Often children notice a dichotomy between what they are taught in the classroom and real life. They are taught healthy living patterns but are served unhealthy lunches and are provided little opportunity for aerobic exercise. Instruction is given in self-responsibility, but the family culture teaches passivity in self-care."

Incorporated in both the areas of education and environment are the experiences and influences which provide motivation for initial change. The Louis Harris survey (1983) noted major factors which lead adults to improve their health habits: a growing self-awareness, the advice and situation of another. The most frequently mentioned influence was awareness due to the media or educational classes. This suggests that education campaigns, along with a supportive environment, can be successful in promoting preventive lifestyle changes.

Self-Esteem

Self-esteem has been defined by K.J. Gergen (1971) as "the extent to which the person feels positive about himself." Self-esteem strongly affects whether an individual continues with or drops out of an exercise program. Self-esteem is a critical matter not only for the overweight, the smoker, the depressed, and the hostile, but for the "average" person as well.

To foster self-esteem through a program of exercise, a positive program with supportive leaders is needed. As Dr. Philip Wilson stated, "If you have the choice between a big budget, great facilities, or a good staff, always pick a good staff. That is what will keep the participants coming" (1984). This is where traditional physical education has failed. For too long, physical education departments have concerned themselves with building athletes, not fit students, and with clean locker rooms rather than clean arteries. As Kuntzleman (1982) has stated, "Too often, physical education has been punitive. Rather, it should and can be fun, something children can participate in not only now, but when they are 30, 40, 50, or beyond. Competition bruises egos and does not foster continued participation."

As previously stated, overweight individuals are frequent dropouts. Much of this is related to their self-esteem. In *The Feelin' Good Youth Fitness Report* (Kuntzleman & Drake, 1984), it was found among children that there is a strong inverse correlation between skinfold levels and self-esteem (Table 1). This was especially true for girls. Even girls with average body fat had significantly lower self-esteem scores than leaner girls. Boys with high levels of body fat had significantly lower scores than other boys.

Following the intervention of Feelin' Good, an aerobic-based cardiovascular health program, significant decreases in skinfold levels and significant increases in self-esteem were found among these same children (Kuntzleman & Drake, 1984). Significant increases were also found in the categories of self-image, fate, and their comparisons of selves to others. These all make for increased program adherence.

Goals and Values

Goals are important in all aspects of life, especially fitness. Goals provide impetus to stay with a program of exercise. Working toward a particular end point makes an activity more enjoyable. Setting goals in the business world is an expected, cost-effective practice. Programs of fitness also should aid participants in establishing and realizing their personal goals.

The process of setting goals, however, often seems laborious, and the setting of unrealistic goals can have negative consequences. As Kuntzleman (1981) has stated, "As we mature past elementary years, we often feel our imagination is destroyed. Along with Santa Claus, the Tooth Fairy, and the Easter Bunny, we throw out our own hopes and dreams." We need to help children establish goals early in life so that they will know how to establish goals, have something to work towards, and have the

Table 1 Comparison of Skinfold Fitness Classifications and Self-Esteem of Feelin' Good® and Control Groups (Pretest Data)

Skinfolds	n	Self-Image	Fate	Good as Others	Well-Adjusted	Locus of Control	Combined Score
Very poor	41	2.71	2.04	2.20	2.40	2.38	2.37
Poor	96	2.81[a]	1.92	2.35[a]	2.45	2.47	2.45[a]
Average	141	2.80[a]	1.87	2.34[a]	2.45	2.46	2.44[a]
Good	88	2.82[A]	1.89	2.41[A]	2.50[a,h]	2.47	2.48[A,h]
Excellent	43	2.87[A,h]	1.92	2.49[A,b,c]	2.53[a,g,h]	2.43	2.52[A,c,g]

Significance

a [A]Significant in comparison to Very Poor

b [B]Significant in comparison to Poor

c [C]Significant in comparison to Average

d [D]Significant in comparison to Good

a type: < 05.

A type: < 01.

Trends

[g] Trend in comparison to Very Poor

[g] Trend in comparison to Poor

[h] Trend in comparison to Average

skills to continue to develop goals throughout life. Children need the opportunity to daydream and use their imagination for the future.

John Goddard was such a child. At age 15, John made a list of things he wanted to do with his life. He set 127 goals! Among these were to climb Mt. Everest, explore the Nile, explore the Great Barrier Reef of Australia, write a book, circumnavigate the globe, and read the entire *Encyclopedia Brittanica*. Idle dreaming, you may say. However, at last report, John Goddard, age 57, had accomplished 108 of his 127 goals. Still to go: to visit all 141 countries of the world (he has been to only 113 so far), live to see the twenty-first century (he'll be 75), and visit the moon.

Not all children are as adventurous as John Goddard. Yet, goals should be established for each category of life—emotional, nutritional, interpersonal, mental, spiritual, and physical. Guidance is needed to set realistic goals. The children also need to realize that goals may be changed with time. Short-term, intermediate, and long-term goals should be established for each category. Short-term goals should be posted, the long-term ones filed for future reference.

This process of setting goals aids in establishing self-responsibility, whereby children are not forced by others to change, but are allowed to guide his or her own life. Goals give children something to work for. Goals help children realize that they themselves are responsible for whom and what they become.

Goal setting goes hand in hand with establishing values. Values, the basic beliefs held about what is "good" and what "ought to be," greatly influence what people do (Kuntzleman, 1978). Values are often subconsciously developed through the influence and examples of others. Yet, children need the opportunity to examine their own values and practice personal decision making. This process will help children become more committed, acting on their values more consciously and effectively.

Enjoyment

Enjoyment is last on this list, but is probably the most important factor in adherence to a program of exercise.

Americans are pleasure-seeking, going to great extremes to find new sources of fun. In the past, exercise and fitness have largely been left out of this search for pleasure because of the punitive approach presented. However, researchers continually document both psychological and physiological benefits of aerobic-based exercise. Thus, shouldn't exercise be sought for pleasure?

Schools, however, have turned children away from exercise with the punitive approach of traditional physical education: Missed baskets result in running laps, losers do push-ups, and there's the "no pain, no gain" philosophy. This approach has prompted children to turn to other avenues for pleasure—avenues as detrimental as drugs and alcohol.

It has been stated that work is what we have to do but leisure is what we want to do. Children can learn to like activity, but a positive, non-threatening, noncompetitive approach is needed. Programs must be fun, involve a variety of activities, and provide enough exercise to promote cardiovascular health.

Conclusion

To provide motivation for a lifetime of involvement in exercise, exercise participants must (a) receive proper education within a wellness philosophy, (b) be provided with a supportive environment, (c) be aided in developing better self-esteem, (d) set goals and develop values, and (e) find enjoyment. These principles apply to both children and adults. Employment of these principles will help participants feel good about themselves and about life in general.

In providing children or adults a program for exercise or anything else, it must be realized that not every person becomes actively involved. However, as the Feelin' Good film (Kuntzleman, 1982) states, "We do not leave the intellectual, spiritual, or emotional needs of our children to chance. Why should we leave their physical needs to chance?" Let's motivate and provide our children with the opportunity for a lifetime of fun and fitness.

References

Brownell, K.D., & Stunkard, A.J. (1980). Physical activity in the development and control of obesity. In A.J. Stunkard (Ed.), *Obesity* (pp. 67-77). Philadelphia: Saunders.

Buffone, G.W., Sachs, M.L., & Dowd, E.T. (1979). *Cognitive-behavioral strategies for facilitating maintenance of exercise behavior.* Unpublished manuscript.

Dishman, R.K. (1984, October). Prescription for exercise adherence. In K. Palmer (Chair), *Cardiac rehabilitation, exercise testing, and prescription.* Symposium conducted at the La Crosse Health and Sports Science Symposium, La Crosse, WI.

Dishman, R.K., Ickes, W.J., & Morgan, W.P. (1980). Self-motivation and adherence to habitual physical activity. *Journal of Applied Social Psychology, 10,* 115,131.

Franklin, B.Z. (1978). Motivating and teaching adults to exercise: Practical suggestions to increase interest and enthusiasm. *Journal of Physical Education and Recreation, 48,* 13-17.

Gergen, K.J. (1971). *The concept of self*. New York: Holt, Rinehart, and Winston.

Harris, Louis, and Associates, Inc. (1983). *Prevention in America: Steps people take—or fail to take—for better health* (survey conducted for *Prevention* magazine).

Ho, P., Graham, L., Blair, S., Wood, P., Haskell, W., Williams, P., Terry, R., & Farquhar, J. (1981, August). *Adherence prediction and pyschological changes following a one-year randomized exercise program*. Paper presented at meeting of the American Psychological Association, Los Angeles.

Keefe, F.J., & Blumenthal, J.A. (1980). The life fitness program: A behavioral approach to making exercise a habit. *Journal of Behavior Therapy and Experimental Psychiatry*, **11**, 31-34.

Kuntzleman, C.T. (1978). *Values strategies for fitness*. Spring Arbor, MI: Arbor Press.

Kuntzleman, C.T. (1981). *Maximum personal energy*. Emmaus, PA: Rodale Press.

Kuntzleman, C.T. (1982). *Feelin' Good film*. Spring Arbor, MI: Fitness Finders.

Kuntzleman, C.T., & Drake, D.A. (1984). *The Feelin' Good youth fitness report*. Spring Arbor, MI: Fitness Finders.

Martin, J.E., Katell, A.D., Webster, J.S., Zegman, M., & Blount, R. (1981, November). *The effects of feedback, reinforcement, and goal selection on exercise adherence*. Paper presented at the meeting of the Association for Advancement of Behavior Therapy, Toronto.

Martin, J.E., & Smith, P.O. (1981, November). *Factors predicting exercise adherence: A two-year evaluation*. Paper presented at the meeting of the Association for Advancement of Behavior Therapy, Toronto.

Olson, J.M., & Zanna, M.P. (1982). *Predicting adherence to a program of physical exercise: an empirical study*. Toronto, Ontario: Ministry of Tourism and Recreation.

Perrin, B. (1979). Survey of physical activity in the regional municipality of Waterloo. *Recreation Research Review*, **6**, 48-52.

Sticking with fitness. (1982). Toronto, Ontario: Ministry of Tourism and Recreation.

Thompson, C.E., & Wankel, L.M. (1980). The effects of perceived activity choice upon frequency of exercise behavior. *Journal of Applied Social Psychology*, **10**, 436-443.

Those who know but don't do. (1982). Toronto, Ontario: Ministry of Tourism and Recreation, Fitness Ontario.

Wankel, L.M. (1979). Motivating involvement in adult physical activity programs. *Recreation Research Review*, **66**, 40-43.

Wankel, L.M. (1981, August). *Social psychological dimensions of physical activity involvement*. Paper presented at the Canadian Congress on Leisure Research, Edmonton, Alberta.

Webster's new universal unabridged dictionary (2nd ed.). (1979). New York: Simon & Schuster.

Wilson, P.K. (1984, October). Administrative concerns: Preventative and rehabilitative exercise programs. In W. Kaufman (Chair), *Cardiac rehabilitation, exercise testing, and prescription*. Symposium conducted at the La Crosse Health and Sports Science Symposium, La Crosse, WI.

Chapter 4

Behavioral Barriers to Health-Related Physical Fitness

Rod K. Dishman

Clinical experiences in adult exercise programs reveal exceptions to the general principles governing fitness training that can have great importance for individual participants. This chapter describes instances when health-related outcomes of fitness testing and training can be influenced by factors that are largely psychological or behavioral in nature. I will give examples of how the study of behavioral fitness—behavioral and psychological factors in health-related exercise—can help clarify the role of fitness training in preventive medicine and public health. Three types of behavioral barriers to fitness will be addressed: (a) motivational factors that interact with standard exercise training prescriptions to influence compliance, (b) psychological and behavioral factors that might influence the meaning of diagnostic and prescriptive clinical exercise stress tests, and (c) emotional factors that can influence physiological and medical adaptations to submaximal exercise training. My goal is to present an empirical case that the implementation of existing standards for adult fitness programming at times fails to optimize health-related outcomes if it is exclusively based on physiological principles and ignores behavioral factors that can influence both health and fitness.

Prescriptions for Fitness and Health

Conventional training guidelines (American College of Sports Medicine, 1978) for insuring relatively risk-free gains in cardiopulmonary fitness are well supported by an empirical literature. The magnitude of anticipated increases in fitness (defined by objective standards such as $\dot{V}O_2$ maximum) can be reliably estimated for different age groups and for different levels of initial fitness if the type, intensity, duration, and frequency of the exercise stimulus to be used is specified. This knowledge has greatly advanced the implementation of systematic fitness plans that are effective and safe for large numbers of participants.

Exercise scientists and clinicians in fitness programs recognize, however, that some participants do not respond as expected. Existing principles of training have limitations in their ability to predict several outcomes that are related to health. As the longstanding interest in the relationship between fitness and health has accelerated in recent years (Mason & Powell, 1985), it has become clear that adaptations to exercise and physical activity that bear on decreased risk for chronic diseases, premature mortality, and increased mental health may at times be different from those that lead to greater functional capacity (Dishman, 1988). Convincing epidemiologic studies support that moderate to high physical activity levels (1000-2000 calories per week above routine expenditures) appear causally linked to lowered risk for morbidity and mortality due to heart disease and other chronic disorders (Paffenbarger, Hyde, Wing, & Steinmetz, 1984).

However, studies showing that fitness level, more so than activity, offers a unique health protection are less compelling (Blair et al., 1983; Cooper et al., 1976; Gibbons, Blair, Cooper, & Smith, 1983). Fitness increases can be accompanied by reductions in such major risk factors for disease as weight, blood pressure, and stress emotions, and by improved serum lipoprotein fractions (Dishman, 1985; Siscovick, LaPorte, & Newman, 1985). However, the same outcomes can also be seen for some individuals following increased physical activity of moderate intensities generally too low to induce significant increases in fitness as measured by conventional standards (e.g., $\dot{V}O_2$ maximum). Fitness can also increase without being accompanied by reductions in risk factors. A study that directly ties increased fitness with decreased disease morbidity or mortality or with increased mental health is virtually nonexistent. While the balance of evidence indeed supports that fitness and health are closely aligned for a large portion of the population (Powell & Paffenbarger, 1985), each result reflects unique and independent antecedent and consequent conditions and is measured in different ways. See Table 1 (Caspersen, Powell, & Christenson, 1985).

The differences between health, fitness, and physical activity have important implications for exercise programming. One is that many individuals may be able to increase their health through increased activity at lower intensities than required for high-level fitness. Haskell, Montoye, and Orenstein (1985) have suggested that the segments of the population whose health stands to benefit the most from increased activity are the sedentary and low active, more so than those already moderately or highly fit. This benefit can apparently be accomplished by such relatively

Table 1   Elements of Physical Activity and Exercise

Physical Activity	Exercise
1. bodily movement via skeletal muscles	1. bodily movement via skeletal muscles
2. results in energy expenditure	2. results in energy expenditure
3. energy expenditure (kilocalories) varies continuously from low to high	3. energy expenditure (kilocalories) varies continuously from low to high
4. positive correlation with physical fitness	4. very strong positive correlation with physical fitness
	5. planned, structured, and repetitive bodily movement
	6. objective of improving or maintaining physical fitness component(s)

Note. From "Physical Activity, Exercise, and Physical Fitness: Definitions and Distinctions for Health-Related Research" by C.J. Caspersen, K.E. Powell, & G.M. Christenson, 1985, *Public Health Reports,* **100**, p. 127. Copyright 1985 by U.S. Department of Health and Human Service. Adapted by permission.

low-intensity activities as walking, climbing, moderate biking, swimming, and aerobic games. Acceptance of moderate exertion as the fitness norm may be effective not only to meet medical indications for some who are physically impaired, but for motivating people currently sedentary (40% of American adults), among whom 45-65% have no intention of adopting a vigorous fitness regime (Dishman, Sallis, & Orenstein, 1985). Figure 1 represents the direct and indirect relationships between physical activity and disease (Blair, Jacobs, & Powell, 1985).

Programming for Adherence

Recent estimates reveal that only 10-20% of American adults participate in fitness activities with sufficient intensity and regularity to satisfy conventional training guidelines for fitness (Centers for Disease Control, 1985). Only 20-30% of eligible employees will routinely utilize worksite fitness facilities (Shephard, in press), while less than half the users do so at fitness-inducing levels (Fielding, 1982). Likewise, in supervised exercise programs for preventive medicine, it is common for one-half of the participants to drop out prematurely and for exercise prescription com-

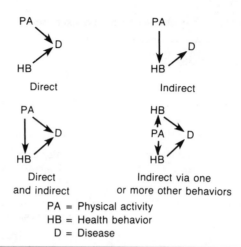

Direct

Indirect

Direct
and indirect

Indirect via one
or more other behaviors

PA = Physical activity
HB = Health behavior
D = Disease

Figure 1 Associations between physical activity and disease may be direct, indirect, or both. *Note.* From "Relationships Between Exercise or Physical Activity and Other Health Behaviors" by S.N. Blair, D.R. Jacobs, and K.E. Powell, 1985, *Public Health Reports*, **100**, p. 178. Copyright 1985 by U.S. Department of Health and Human Services. Reprinted by permission.

pliance among regular attenders to vary from 30-80% (Oldridge, 1982). These findings reveal that existing fitness standards and prescriptions present excessive behavioral challenges for large portions of adults.

Although results of the Ontario Exercise Heart Collaborative Study (OEHCS) (Oldridge et al., 1983) suggest that compliance among post-myocardial infarction patients is no better for low-intensity, low-frequency exercise (1 day per week at less than 50% $\dot{V}O_2$ max) when compared with fitness-increasing activity (3-5 days per week at 60-80% $\dot{V}O_2$ max), studies with obese adolescents and adults, and middle-aged and elderly subjects of normal weight, typically indicate higher compliance with lower intensity prescriptions (Dishman, Sallis, & Orenstein, 1985). Adults who lack positive attitudes toward controlling their health and do not view exercise as a healthy behavior are likely to select low-frequency, low-intensity exercise when given the choice (Sidney & Shepard, 1976), and tend to drop out of intensive fitness programs (Dishman & Gettman, 1980). The sedentary are also apt to view exercise as requiring too much time and effort (Canada Fitness Survey, 1983; George Gallup Organization, 1984), and they report excessive subjective fatigue even when exercise intensity is adjusted for fitness level (Hughes, Crow, Jacobs, Mittlemark, & Leon, 1985). Even among the sedentary who intend to increase their activity, roughly one-half will fail to do so. Perceptions of excessive time and exertion demands (Godin, Shephard, & Colantonio, 1986) and lack of confidence about the ability to carry out a fitness program (Sallis, Haskell, Fortmann, et al., 1986) are common barriers.

These findings imply that the optimal volume of exercise for promoting adherence and health outcomes remains to be identified. Not only may rigid fitness prescriptions be too behaviorally challenging for some (Martin et al., 1984), they may not be biologically necessary. Indeed, a recent study (Epstein, Wing, Koeske, Ossip, & Beck, 1982), that compared a fitness regime with increased activity in daily lifestyle routines (e.g., movement games, walking instead of riding, etc.) found that weight loss among obese adolescents due to increased routine activity was maintained longer than weight loss induced by the fitness regime. Epidemiologic studies showing a health protection effect from exercise have usually defined physical activity by overall caloric expenditure per unit of time. Thus, the health significance of fitness thresholds remains unclear. Because other study suggests that self-choice of activity can increase exercise adherence (Thompson & Wankel, 1980), a more expanded view of what is an appropriate set of activity types, intensities, frequencies, and durations may be justified on behavioral and epidemiologic grounds.

In certain patient groups, restricted prescription may still be needed to reduce cardiopulmonary or orthopedic risks. However, it has long been recognized by clinical experts that there are many plans that can achieve similar fitness outcomes. Recently Haskell, Montoye, and Orenstein (1985) have recommended a minimum expenditure of 4 calories per kilogram of body weight per exercise session for the previously sedentary. Years ago fitness pioneer Bruno Balke (1974) suggested that a total caloric cost per activity session equalling 10% of a person's daily metabolic expenditure provides an effective standard within which various specific plans can be prudently implemented. The motivational importance of encouraging variety has also been recognized for some time (Oldridge, 1977). It is likely, though, that the information given to or perceived by the public about fitness planning, as well as the prescriptions actually implemented in supervised settings, are frequently overly restrictive.

Although existing guidelines for fitness planning (American College of Sports Medicine, 1978) offer ranges rather than specific goals for intensity (60-90% of maximum heart rate or 50-85% of $\dot{V}O_2$ max), duration (15-60 minutes), and frequency (3-5 days per week), it is a common clinical observation that many inactive individuals who regard exercise as too effortful or time-consuming have rather narrow and fixed views of what is desirable or worthwhile exercise. These views are frequently too low or too high.

Representative population surveys reveal that many believe their current patterns of very low intensity or low frequency exertion are adequate for fitness and health (George Gallup Organization, 1984; Perrier Study, 1979; Presidents Council on Physical Fitness and Sports, 1973). In instances where existing motivation is adequate, increased knowledge about minimum requirements for fitness could alter exercise patterns.

An equally common perception is that only a single plan for fitness is effective, though this may exceed a person's preferences for activity type, intensity, periodicity, or setting. This is akin to the well-known abstainer's fallacy in various behavior changes (e.g., dieting, smoking, and alcohol cessation), with an all-or-nothing mentality that only complete restriction to a single plan and perfect discipline can be effective. Too often the plan adopted far exceeds a person's behavioral skills. This can lead to a self-fulfilling prophecy of failure when a single backslide is misperceived or falsely projected as a forecast for total relapse. The likelihood of this seems reinforced by conventional fitness concepts and practices that set exercise targets or thresholds in plans for fitness gains. Study shows (Martin et al., 1984) that specific, fixed, long-term exercise goals are motivating, but daily goals require flexibility if adherence is to be increased in persons with low self-motivation.

The past assumption that noncompliers must always be changed to fit the fitness program may need to be reversed to better fit the program to the participant. For some, non-high-fitness activities can be appropriate for both health and behavioral compliance. Aside from lowering the risk of orthopedic injuries and sudden death due to heavy exertion (Siscovick, LaPorte, & Newman, 1985), exercise prescriptions that modify mode and intensity may facilitate participation among some individuals in a way that more than compensates for any lessening of potential fitness gains (Pollock, 1988). Population-based study (Sallis et al., 1986) shows that more than twice as many adults will adopt a new routine of moderate activity (e.g., walking) than adopt a fitness regime. Women are six times as likely to choose a walking program than are men.

Modifying physiological guidelines for training in order to serve behavioral needs seems justified also by the results from clinical exercise trials that conflict over the importance of fitness compliance in the prevention of morbidity and mortality due to ischemic heart disease (Rechnitzer et al., 1983; Sanne, 1973; Shephard, Corey, & Kavanagh, 1981). Indeed, research in behavioral medicine suggests compliance with any medical prescription can exert a healthful effect independent of the medical outcome of the compliance (Epstein, 1984). Finding the optimal exercise prescription for compliance and health gains has received less research attention, and may be a more difficult challenge, than prescriptions for fitness. For these reasons, it remains an important area for study in adult fitness.

Behavioral Problems With Intensity Prescriptions

The general problem of exercise compliance is addressed in more detail in chapter 5 and elsewhere (Dishman, Sallis, & Orenstein, 1985; Martin

& Dubbert, 1985a). However, it is important also to recognize that participants can adhere to an exercise program (i.e., attend the recommended number of sessions for the specified amount of time) but fail to comply with the prescribed intensity. Also, the intensity prescription may at times be behaviorally inappropriate. Intensity prescriptions have particular significance not only because they influence cardiovascular risks among some patient groups and determine fitness adaptations, but because they can be aversive and create barriers to motivation. Increases in a person's exertion level seem more resistive to interventions than do increases in frequency or duration. Studies using behavioral modification techniques to increase physical activity have focused more on frequency or duration of exercise than intensity or type, and the increases seen in weekly caloric expenditure have typically been less than half that believed necessary to reduce health risk (Dishman et al., 1985).

Two specific behavioral aspects of exercise intensity prescription bear on compliance concerns and have clinical significance. The first stems from the behavioral impact of physiological inaccuracies that can occur when prescribing a training heart rate range based on either measured or age-predicted heart rate reserve. The second involves both random and motivated errors that reduce compliance with typical training intensity prescriptions once they are given.

Limitations of the Training Heart Rate

Various indicators of exertional strain can be used for exercise intensity prescriptions (e.g., caloric cost, percentage of $\dot{V}O_2$ maximum, ventilatory or lactate breakpoints), but heart rate is the most practically feasible and widespread. Heart rate prescriptions present some problems, though. Even when variability due to age, training status, and testing mode is accounted for, idiosyncratic differences in measured heart rate maximum (HR max) remain that are of clinical significance (Londeree & Moeschberger, 1982). When the more common procedure of age-predicted HR max (220 beats per minute [bpm] minus age) is used, even greater problems can occur. Errors of 15 bpm above or below a true maximum can be expected in 3 of 10 cases (Wilson, 1977). Heart rate is also altered by emotional states and medications.

For these reasons, exclusive reliance on heart rate for testing and prescription can lead to overestimates and underestimates of optimal metabolic strain for some individuals. For example, a conservative intensity prescription of 60% of age-predicted HR reserve for a 50-year-old with a resting pulse of 70 bpm [([(220 bpm − 50) − 70 bpm] • 0.60) + 70 bpm] yields a training heart rate of 130 bpm. On average this approximates a metabolic strain of 60% $\dot{V}O_2$ max. In 3 of 10 cases, however, if this prescription were based on a measured heart rate maximum, a training heart rate ranging from 121 bpm to 139 bpm would result. This means that when a single age-predicted prescription rule is used with everyone, in 30% of the cases the possible intensity prescribed for training could range as low as 65% to as high as 90% of actual maximum heart rate. In 5% of the cases, the true maximum heart rate would range from 140 bpm to 200 bpm and the training prescription could be as low as 56% or as high as 95% of HR max. Although these levels remain close to ACSM guidelines for groups, clearly, an appropriate metabolic intensity can be grossly misjudged for some people using procedures that are typical in many adult fitness programs.

Because perceived exertion is more closely linked with relative heart rate and relative oxygen consumption than with absolute heart rate (Pandolph, 1983), the subjective strain also should vary widely. Hence, it is not surprising that participants given age-predicted heart ranges frequently complain they are too easy or too hard.

Several exercise clinicians (Bruce, DeRoven, & Hossack, 1980; Burke & Collins, 1984; Chow & Wilmore, 1984; Pollock, 1988) have suggested using ratings of perceived exertion (RPE) as a complement to heart rate prescriptions. Reports show that RPE can be a better estimate of $\dot{V}O_2$ max than HR alone (Noble, Maresh, & Richey, 1981), and that a prediction model combining HR and RPE is a better measure of voluntary working capacity than either measure alone (Morgan & Borg, 1976). However, studies of how the two might be weighted to optimize a metabolic training prescription are not available. See Figure 2 for an illustration of perceived exertion and relative exercise intensity during treadmill exercise (Hanson, 1984).

Borg (1973) earlier proposed that the model RPE × 10 = HR could be effective, but several clinicians (Burke & Collins, 1984; Hanson, 1984; Pollock, 1988) each report clinical observations that a correction factor of 20-30 bpm must be added (i.e., [RPE × 10] + 20 to 30 bpm = HR) for RPEs of 11-13 and heart rates within typical training ranges of 130-160 bpm. Similarly, Burke and Collins (1984) have observed among experienced adult joggers that RPEs of 11-16 correspond to heart rates ranging from 144-174 in healthy adults from about 16-50 years of age. Because study has shown that subjects can reproduce a treadmill pace using previous RPEs when HRs were 150 bpm or above and RPEs were 12 or higher (Smutok, Skrinar, & Pandolf, 1980), perceived exertion holds practical promise for improving intensity prescriptions among some people.

This is reinforced by a recent study (Dwyer & Bybee, 1983) of 20 untrained college women. On bicycle ergometry, 9 subjects exceeded ventilatory threshold at 75% of HR reserve. This increased to 13 and 15 subjects at 80% and 85%, respectively, of HR reserve or, correspondingly, 70% and 75% of $\dot{V}O_2$ max. Because 75% of HR reserve is a widespread intensity prescription for college women, these findings suggest that excessive strain can frequently result when it is employed with untrained subjects as seen in Tables 2 and 3 (Dwyer & Bybee, 1983). This is sup-

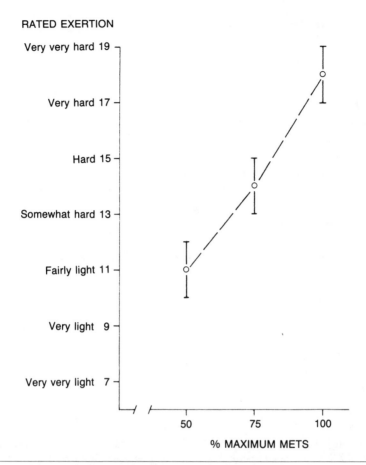

Figure 2 Perceived exertion (mean ± standard deviation) and relative exercise intensity during treadmill exercise (% maximum METs). The linear relationship between exertion rating and the percent of maximum exercise capacity provides a useful monitoring end point for exercise testing. *Note.* From "Clinical Exercise Testing" by P. Hanson, 1984, in R. Strauss (Ed.), *Sports Medicine* (p. 24), Philadelphia: W.B. Saunders. Copyright 1984 by W.B. Saunders Company. Reprinted by permission.

ported by the observation by Purvis and Cureton (1981) that ventilatory threshold is associated with RPEs of 13 to 14. A rating of 13 corresponds with a subjective category of "somewhat hard." It seems unlikely that sedentary individuals will find intensities markedly above ventilatory or lactate thresholds reinforcing. See Figure 3 (Chow & Wilmore, 1984).

Problems of Self-Regulation

There are also random and motivated errors when a prescribed training heart rate range is self-regulated by the patient. Chow and Wilmore (1984)

Table 2 Anaerobic Threshold and Heart Rate

% HR Reserve	60	65	70	75	80	85	90
Mean HR	140	145	151	156	162	167	173
Subjects above AT[a]	1	3	5	9	13	15	20
Subjects below AT	19	17	15	11	7	5	0

[a]Number of subjects above/below AT at 60-90% HR reserve.

Note. From J. Dwyer and R. Bybee, "Heart Rate Indices of the Anaerobic Threshold," *Medicine and Science in Sports and Exercise*, Volume 15, p. 74, © by The American College of Sports Medicine, 1983.

Table 3 Anaerobic Threshold and Heart Rate % $\dot{V}O_2$ Max

% $\dot{V}O_2$ Max	60	65	70	75	80
Mean $\dot{V}O_2$	1.33	1.44	1.55	1.67	1.78
Subjects above AT[a]	1	4	13	15	19
Subjects below AT	19	16	7	5	1
% HR	78.5	82.5	86.0	90.0	94.0

[a]Number of subjects above AT at 60-80% $\dot{V}O_2$ max.

Note. From J. Dwyer and R. Bybee, "Heart Rate Indices of the Anaerobic Threshold," *Medicine and Science in Sports and Exercise*, Volume 15, p. 74, © by The American College of Sports Medicine, 1983.

found that during four daily 15-minute sessions of self-paced treadmill jogging without feedback, adult males were able to remain in their prescribed training range (60-70% $\dot{V}O_2$ max) only 25% of the time. Allowing subjects to periodically monitor pulse rate increased accuracy to a still-low 55%, while using RPE gave an accuracy of 48.5%. Average error for the heart rate monitoring group was just 2.6 bpm above the prescribed group mean, and error for RPE was 5 bpm below. However, 60% of control subjects receiving the prescription instructions typical of adult fitness programs exercised at a mean heart rate during each session that was outside their individually prescribed ranges. See Figure 3 (Chow & Wilmore, 1984). In our recent study (Dishman et al., 1987) the mean error between prescribed and attained target heart rate (THR) on the first day of jogging, following a typical prescription (60% HR reserve) based on measured heart rate maximum, was +23 bpm. Subjects who had been

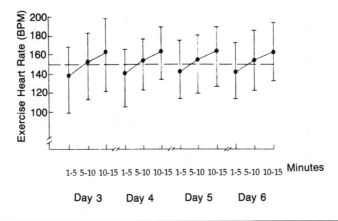

1-5 5-10 10-15 1-5 5-10 10-15 1-5 5-10 10-15 1-5 5-10 10-15 Minutes

Day 3   Day 4   Day 5   Day 6

Figure 3 Mean exercise heart rates for group 3 (no prescription). Training heart rate = 150.8 beats/min; mean = 152.8 beats/min; standard deviation = 9.8; t = 0.3. *Note.* From "The Regulation of Exercise Intensity by Ratings of Perceived Exertion" by R.J. Chow and J.H. Wilmore, 1984, *Journal of Cardiac Rehabilitation,* **4,** p. 385. Copyright 1984 by Le Jacq Publishing. Reprinted by permission.

given RPE instructions during treadmill testing had a mean error of +3 bpm; however, the standard deviation was 19 bpm. This suggests that the prescribed target of 140 bpm could have been behaviorally inappropriate for some subjects. Most subjects who overshot THR were still exercising below 75% of heart rate reserve.

Though little is known about the impact *preferred* levels of exertion have on prescription compliance, it is unlikely that prescriptions based on HR and RPE will optimize compliance for some individuals. Farrell, Gates, Maksud, and Morgan (1982) observed that during continuous treadmill running, trained runners chose to exercise at an intensity approximating 75% of $\dot{V}O_2$ max even though their perceived exertion at this level (11.5 on the Borg scale) was significantly greater than that at 60% $\dot{V}O_2$ max, but not different from 80% $\dot{V}O_2$ max. For these findings see Figure 4 (Farrell, Gates, Maksud, & Morgan, 1982). Beta-endorphin/Beta-lipotropin immunoreactivity was suprisingly greatest at the lowest exercise intensity (60% $\dot{V}O_2$ max). This supports the view that the slower, less-preferred pace was psychologically more stressful to the experienced runner. See Figure 5 (Farrell, Gates, Maksud, & Morgan, 1982).

Collectively, the implication of these studies is that for some individuals the errors seen when target heart rate (THR) is self-regulated may reflect a preference for other intensities and that these may be metabolically more appropriate as well. We are currently examining differences in perceived exertion and ventilatory threshold between low fit, sedentary persons and high fit, active persons when they are allowed to choose their preferred intensity during a continuous exercise session. Our ultimate objectives

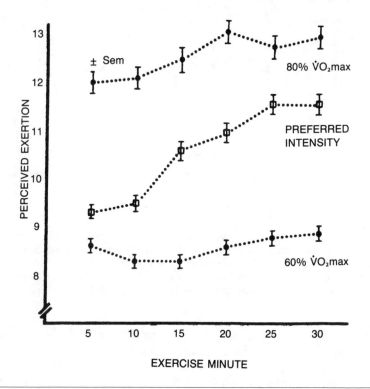

Figure 4   Perceived exertion as assessed by the Borg scale during 30 min of treadmill running at 3 intensities (*n* = 6). *Note*. From "Increases in Plasma B-Endorphin/B-Lipotropin Immunoreactivity After Treadmill Running in Humans" by P.A. Farrell, W.K. Gates, M.G. Maksud, and W.P. Morgan, 1982, *Journal of Applied Physiology*, **52**, p. 1247. Copyright 1982 by The American Physiological Society. Reprinted by permission.

are to determine the impact on program adherence of prescribed training intensities that are outside preferred ranges, and to quantify the metabolic and behavioral significance of modifying prescriptions to better match exertional preferences.

Other studies suggest that some types of individuals are motivated to exceed conventional prescriptions. Gillilan et al. (1984) have found that subjects high in exercise self-efficacy (high confidence in their ability to exercise) tended to overshoot training heart rate prescriptions; this is consistent with common clinical observations that some people are motivated beyond safe levels of exercise. Similarly, Rejeski, Morley, and Miller (1984) have found that cardiac patients scoring high on the Type A and job involvement scales of the Jenkins Activity Survey (JAS) trained in the upper range of their HR prescriptions and had greater than expected increases in maximum met level after training, even though they were irregular attendees at the supervised exercise sessions. This is consistent with population-based study in Belgium (Kittel et al., 1983) showing that

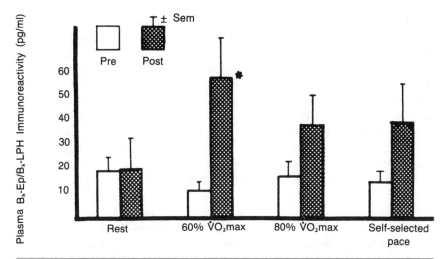

Figure 5   Plasma B_h-Ep/B_h-LPH immunoreactivity (pg/ml) before and after 30 min of treadmill running at 3 intensities (n = 6). *Significantly higher than prevalue at $p < 0.05$. *Note*. From "Increases in Plasma B-Endorphin/ B-Lipotropin Immunoreactivity After Treadmill Running in Humans" by P.A. Farrell, W.K. Gates, M.G. Maksud, and W.P. Morgan, 1982, *Journal of Applied Physiology, 52*, p. 1247. Copyright 1982 by The American Physiological Society. Reprinted by permission.

Type A males tend to exercise at high weekly energy levels during leisure time whereas Type Bs are low active. In a sample of 49 middle-aged males (Dishman, Holly, & Schelegle, 1985), we saw a strong correlation between our self-motivation scale and both the Type A and hard-driving scales of the JAS. Only self-motivation was correlated with self-limited treadmill performance. Because self-motivation frequently predicts exercise adherence (Dishman, Sallis, & Orenstein, 1985), these findings suggest that it is the achievement motivation aspects of Type A that influence exercise behavior. Although intrinsic motivation to train at high intensity can increase cardiovascular and orthopedic risks, high exertion personalities may be useful models for understanding exercise reinforcers that might increase exertion in the sedentary. Within medically safe limits, exercise compliance among some participants may be increased if intensity prescriptions for them are made less conservative.

Prescribing From Treadmill Performance

Because of the potential risks of ventricular tachycardia and sudden cardiac death during maximum exertion in some aged and patient populations (Siscovick et al., 1985), and due to the practical difficulties in invoking a plateau in oxygen consumption for untrained or unmotivated subjects, most clinical graded exercise tests are stopped by an attending physician or by the subject due to subjective symptoms of fatigue, angina, or pro dromal signs (e.g., aberrant beats) that suggest increasing cardiovascular risk. Because one major goal in exercise stress testing is frequently not the determination of a true $\dot{V}O_2$ max, but the determination of an exertion level that appears cardiovascularly safe, symptom-limited tests are usually appropriate. They do present problems for some subjects, however. Many test protocols establish such a prior cutoff for a clinically maximum test as 75-85% of age-predicted maximum heart rate. If risk signs permit this intensity to be attained, the test is considered sufficiently stressful to be of diagnostic value for estimating the likelihood of myocardial ischemia or other abnormal cardiovascular functions. The predictive accuracy of age-predicted heart rate and of biomedical indicators of exertional strain is sufficiently unreliable, however, that many physicians also rely on subjective patient symptoms for interpreting overall patient stress at each work stage. Self-report scales for angina pectoris (Borg, 1962) and scales for perceived exertion, such as Borg's category-rating scale (1973) are now common fixtures at most stress-testing stations. This shows that despite technical precision in modern cardiology, exercise testing retains a substantial component of clinical judgment. This subjective aspect of exercise stress testing is often a useful complement to objective biomedical assessments. It also can permit significant errors for some people, though.

It is a clinical observation, reproduced in many laboratories, that as many as 1 in 10 adults appear to suppress ratings of fatigue below those expected for a given heart rate or proportion of $\dot{V}O_2$ max. If test termination is influenced by those subjective symptoms, an inflated exercise prescription intensity might result. Although the testing physician is not likely to permit this to exceed heart rates that interrupt a normal sinus rhythm, undetected risks may still be present or may be exaggerated during actual training sessions where other cardiovascular stresses (e.g., daily hassles or competitive excitement during group games) may be exaggerated. Similarly, it is clinically clear that some patients are motivated by the testing environment to push to performance limits that can exceed medically safe levels.

Because Type A individuals are believed to show exaggerated motivation and to suppress subjective fatigue when challenged by achievement- or goal-directed settings, several studies have examined performance differences between Type A and Type B individuals during treadmill testing. Carver, Coleman, and Glass (1976) observed that 10 college males classified as As on the student version of the Jenkins Activity Survey (JAS) self-selected a higher percentage of $\dot{V}O_2$ max during a sham Balke endurance test and reported less subjective fatigue than 11 Type Bs who were otherwise matched. Rejeski, Morley, and Miller (1983) reported a canonical correlation between JAS sub-scales and maximum respiratory exchange ratio (RER) during a multistage treadmill test in 44 male cardiac patients. RPE max was unrelated, however, to either RER or JAS. In another study of outpatient males (n = 43) (Castell & Blumenthal, 1984), JAS Type As had longer treadmill time than Bs during a symptom-limited, graded test, but did not differ in subjective fatigue or pain during the test. Although As and Bs did not differ in maximum heart rate or coronary artery disease, no data on $\dot{V}O_2$ max were presented. Thus, relative strain of the exercise could not be compared. No differences in objective and subjective treadmill responses were seen between a small group (n = 11) of female As and Bs.

Conversely, in two similar experiments with middle-aged males in a preventive exercise program (n = 43), Ross, Morgan, and Leventhal (1978) found no difference in ratings of perceived exertion (RPE) during a Balke test between As and Bs, classified either by structured interview or JAS. Likewise, no RPE difference between As and Bs (n = 60) was found during a 30-minute bicycle ride at 100 watts. Among 40 post-MI middle-aged males, Type As (n = 27) and Type Bs (n = 13) (identified by structured interview) did not differ in completed stages (100 kpm increments each minute) during a standardized bicycle ergometer endurance test or on RPE throughout the test (Schlegel, Wellwood, Copps, Gruchow, & Sharratt, 1980). In our recent study of 49 asymptomatic adult males (Dishman, Holly, & Schelegle, 1985), we also saw no relationships between JAS scores, RPE, and either self-selected submaximal (60-80% VO_2 max) or symptom-limited VO_2 max during a graded treadmill test.

Results of these studies remain equivocal because different treadmill protocols and end points have been used with homogenous samples from very different populations of subjects. Also, different measures of subjective effort and Type A behavior have been employed. This prevents direct comparisons between studies. To help resolve standardization problems, we are conducting a study of 85 men and 20 women of various ages (25 to 70 years) and fitness levels using three standardized measures of Type A, Borg's perceived exertion scale, and a treadmill protocol that permits both a voluntary selection of a submaximal exercise intensity and a clinically limited "maximum." We are also planning an empirically based strategy whereby individuals who show atypical perceived exertion at standard exercise strain will first be identified, and then described by psychological and behavioral characteristics in addition to Type A that are theoretically linked to fatigue suppression.

Diagnostic Events During Graded Exercise and Training

Studies suggest that psychological and behavioral factors may also influence diagnostic aspects of exercise stress testing. Common clinical observations reveal that some patients (particularly those who are inexperienced) show behavioral (Davis, Gass, & Bassett, 1981) and cardiovascular (e.g., increased HR and blood pressure) signs of anxiety while being prepared for a graded exercise test and during early warm-up stages of the test itself (American College of Sports Medicine, 1978).

Aberrant Beats

Because arrhythmia is the leading cause of sudden cardiac death, one of the goals of exercise stress testing is to determine exercise heart rate intensities where safe exertion can be expected. Also, the evaluative stress associated with diagnostic exercise testing can be different from that accompanying training sessions, so it is important to understand more fully the relationship between mental stress and metabolic stress as they both influence cardiac rhythm. Although the major causes of abnormal electrocardiographic responses to exercise relate to cardiopathology (Hanson, 1984), Reich (1985) has concluded that about 20% of all arrhythmia cases are associated with intense emotions, particularly anger and perceived loss of control. It is believed emotions operate through central nervous system influences to destabilize an already vulnerable heart. See Table 4 (Reich, 1985). Direct regional electrical stimulation of the cerebral cortex and the hypothalamus can precipitate arrhythmia and ventricular fibrillation (Hockman, Mauck, & Hoff, 1966). Reich has noted that ectopic beats are experienced during city driving, public speaking, and standard mental stress tests, but are less frequent during meditation and sleep. He also described the profiles of patients reporting acute emotional crises prior to arrhythmias, and suggested that emotional stress can trigger arrhythmias with less cardiopathy. Vulnerable patients have been shown to have more anxious and depressive personalities than otherwise matched controls. In most instances, emotional disturbances appear to precede cardiac aberrancy by 1-24 hours and are unlikely to be acutely transient. Of particular interest, among 25 vulnerable patients, there were 5 cases of arrhythmias during exercise that followed an emotion-inducing episode. Reich has also reported the clinical observation that ventricular tachycardia seems closely linked to acute anger or fear, whereas ventricular fibrillation appears to follow chronic stress. Although study shows that acute exercise can reduce anxiety states in many people, the impact of resistant stress emotions on acute cardiovascular events has not been identified and warrants study.

As early as 1914 (Levy, 1914), it was shown that when such psychogenic agents as nicotine and epinephrine were injected into cat brain, ventricular arrhythmias resulted. More recently, Verrier and Lown (1984) described a dog model for detecting vulnerability to ventricular fibrillation based on a repetitive extrasystole threshold (RE). In this model, graded electric currents are supplied coincidentally to the T-wave apex of the elec-

Table 4 Distribution of Patients With Ventricular Tachycardia and Fibrillation With Antecedent Psychological Disturbances as a Function of Heart Disease

Disease Factors	Ventricular Fibrillation	Ventricular Tachycardia With Syncope	Ventricular Tachycardia	Total	Average Age (yr) (range)
Coronary artery disease	8	3	1	12	55.3 (35-67)
Other heart disease	2	0	0	2	45 (39-51)
No demonstrable heart disease	6	3	2	11	37.9 (25-50)
Total	16	6	3	25	46.9 (25-67)

Note. From "Psychological Predisposition to Life-Threatening Arrythmias" by P. Reich. Reproduced, with permission, from the Annual Review of Medicine, Volume 36, © 1985 by Annual Reviews Inc.

trocardiogram. Thus, the threshold for extrasystole and subsequent ventricular fibrillation can be specified for corresponding heart rates. It is of clinical significance that when animals that had been administered chest shocks while in a Pavlovian sling were later compared with animals that had rested in undisturbed cages, the former exhibited behavioral signs of anxiety (tremor, salivation), sinus tachycardia, and increased mean arterial pressure. See Figure 6 (Verrier & Lown, 1984). Relocation to the cages eliminated these responses. Yet, a later return to the sling reduced the extrasystole threshold by 41%, indicating that learned anxiety markedly influenced vulnerability for ventricular fibrillation. These authors also described experiments where conditioned anticipation to uncontrollable electric shock and induced aggression by denial of food access have produced 30-50% reductions in extrasystole threshold.

Because (a) these effects were associated with increased plasma catecholamines and could be blocked with either cardiac selective (e.g., metoprolol) or nonselective (e.g., propanolol) beta-adrenergic antagonists; (b) ablation of the stellate ganglia did not diminish the conditioning effect (i.e., catecholamine secretion from the adrenal medulla or innervation from other thoracic ganglia are responsible); and (c) at a constant heart

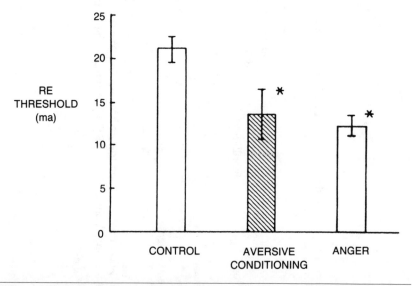

Figure 6 Effects of behavioral stress on the repetitive extrasystole (RE) threshold in eight normal dogs. Both passive aversive conditioning using a mild electric shock and induction of an anger-like state by food-access-denial produced significant reductions in the vulnerable-period threshold. Heart rate was maintained constant during cardiac electrical testing by ventricular pacing. *$p < 0.05$. *Note*. From "Behavioral Stress and Cardiac Arrhythmias" by R.L. Verrier and B. Lown. Reproduced, with permission, from the Annual Review of Physiology, Volume 46, © 1984 by Annual Reviews Inc.

rate, atropine (blocking vagal tone) reduced extrasystole threshold under stressful (high adrenergic state) but not resting (low adrenergic state) conditions, the impact of psychogenic stress on the risk for ventricular fibrillation is confirmed. Figure 7 demonstrates these results (Verrier & Lown, 1984).

The results are consistent with human studies showing that preoperative psychiatric symptoms of Type A behavior are associated with higher risk for ventricular arrhythmias during a 48-hour postoperative period following coronary artery bypass graft surgery, and that preoperative anxiety or depression increased the risk of postoperative atrial arrhythmias (Freeman et al., 1984).

Moreover, it is well known that psychological events increase heart rate (by 10-40 bpm), myocardial contractility, and cardiac output (5 L•min^{-1})

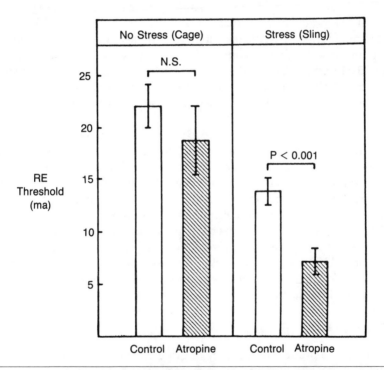

Figure 7   Influence of atropine (0.05 mg•kg^{-1}) on repetitive extrasystole (RE) threshold in conscious dogs exposed to nonaversive and aversive environments. In the aversive setting, blockade of vagal efferent activity with atropine substantially reduced the vulnerable-period threshold, indicating an enhanced propensity for ventricular fibrillation. In the nonstressful setting, where adrenergic activity was low, no effect of the drug was evident. Heart rate was maintained constant during cardiac electrical testing by ventricular pacing. *Note.* From "Behavioral Stress and Cardiac Arrhythmias" by R.L. Verrier and B. Lown. Reproduced, with permission, from the Annual Review of Physiology, Volume 46, © 1984 by Annual Reviews Inc.

at rest (Herd, 1984; Morgan, 1985). This is pronounced during behavioral challenge when task outcomes create conflicts of uncertain controllability or require diligent coping. Individuals can also differ in their responses to these situations. Some may respond to goal-striving or social evaluation situations with increased performance but no cardiovascular reactivity, whereas the converse occurs for others. Imagined emotional states of anger and fear at rest can also increase heart rate by 10 bpm and systolic blood pressure by 6-7 mmHg (Schwartz, Weinberger, & Singer, 1981). Imagining exercise can increase heart rate to 57% of that measured (42 bpm above rest) during 10 minutes of treadmill walking at 3 mph and a 5% grade (Berman, Simonson, & Heron, 1954). During actual exercise of low intensities (e.g., bench stepping or biking at 100 W), imagined emotional states or hypnotic suggestion of increased intensity have similarly increased heart rate (by 12-19 bpm) and systolic blood pressure (by 12-13 mmHg) (Morgan, 1985; Scwartz, Weinberger, & Singer, 1981.). In a related manner, stereotypic relaxation techniques can reduce oxygen consumption by 4-9% during continuous stationary bicycling at heart rates from 95-115 bpm (Benson, Dryer, & Hartley, 1978; Gervino & Veazey, 1984). Similarly, biofeedback procedures can reduce exercise heart rate at submaximal intensities (Goldstein, Ross, & Brady, 1977; Lo & Johnson, 1984; Perski & Engel, 1980).

The practical significance of these experimental findings for clinical testing with patients has not been established. However, it seems likely that the exercise heart rate at which either a normal sinus rhythm is maintained or aberrant beats are seen during the clinical test could be either an overestimate or an underestimate of the true response later seen for training exertion in natural settings. An anxiety response to the treadmill test might falsely limit exertion prescriptions, whereas emotional responses during training (e.g., excitement or anger during games) might render initial HR prescriptions risky. A somewhat analogous circumstance might develop if patients medicated with beta-blockers were tested and trained at different dosages.

S-T Segment Changes

Moreover, the predictive accuracy of graded exercise for detecting myocardial ischemia or coronary heart disease from S-T segment depression is known to vary from very high to very low, depending on the population studied. S-T changes are particularly poor predictors in samples for which prevalence of disease is low. False-positive tests are common in women and in men who are able to exert at high heart rates and systolic blood pressures for their ages (Burke & Collins, 1984; Hanson, 1984). Although little is know about the impact of emotional factors on ECG segmented responses during exercise, there are correlational data suggesting that S-T segment changes during graded exertion are influenced by factors other than increases in myocardial oxygen demand due to increased power output. In one study (Schiffer, Hartley, Schulman, & Abelman, 1976), a 12-minute, graded mental stress quiz was administered to 43 male patients, 33 of whom were corporate executives. Among all subjects, the mean resting baseline heart rate (76 bpm) and blood pressures (136/87 mmHg) increased to 87 bpm and 158/94 mmHg during the mental stress; executives with a history of angina and hypertension showed the greatest increases. During the quiz, 10 of 14 executives with angina had S-T segment depression exceeding .5 mm, 7 exceeded 1.0 mm, and 5 exceeded 1.5 mm. See Figure 8 (Schiffer, Hartley, Schulman, & Abelmann, 1976). Of most interest, among those also taking a graded bicycle exercise stress test, the correlation between S-T depression during mental stress and exercise stress was .63. See Figure 9 (Schiffer, Hartley, Schulman, & Abelmann, 1976).

More recently, Sime, Buell, and Eliot (1980) reported similar changes in blood pressure and heart rate responses to the same graded quiz in male post-MI patients and matched nonpatient controls. In comparison with exercise test results, the emotional stress test induced more premature ventricular contractions but less S-T segment depression. Of related interest, an early one-year training study of post-myocardial infarction executives (Kavanagh, Shephard, Pandit, & Doney, 1970) observed that patients assigned to hypnosis and relaxation therapy showed gains in predicted VO₂ max, resting heart rate, and an elevation in S-T segment depression that were equivalent to matched subjects who exercised once

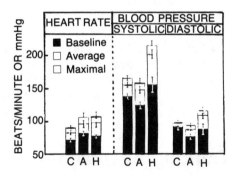

Figure 8 Heart rate and blood pressure in the executive groups; control (C, $n = 19$); angina without hypertension (A, $n = 8$); and angina with a history of hypertension (H, $n = 6$). Values are mean ± 1 standard error. Control values before the quiz (black bars) and average (cross-hatched bars) and maximal (white bars) values during the quiz are indicated. *Note.* From "The Quiz Electrocardiogram: A New Diagnostic and Research Technique for Evaluating the Relation Between Emotional Stress and Ischemic Heart Disease" by F. Schiffer, H.H. Hartley, C.L. Schulman, and W.H. Abelmann, 1976, *American Journal of Cardiology*, **37**, p. 43. Copyright 1976 by Technical Publishing Co. Reprinted by permission.

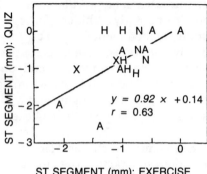

ST SEGMENT (mm): EXERCISE

Figure 9   Maximal S-T segment depression in response to the quiz and to exercise tolerance testing. A = seven executives with angina without a history of hypertension; H = five executives with angina and a history of hypertension; N = three nonexecutives with angina; X = two asymptomatic executives with a positive exercise tolerance test. *Note.* From "The Quiz Electrocardiogram: A New Diagnostic and Research Technique for Evaluating the Relation Between Emotional Stress and Ischemic Heart Disease" by F. Schiffer, H.H. Hartley, C.L. Schulman, and W.H. Abelmann, 1976, *American Journal of Cardiology,* **37**, p. 45. Copyright 1976 by Technical Publishing Company. Reprinted by permission.

per week for 1-1.5 hours. In a similar report on additional patients after a second year, S-T segment changes for the hypnotherapy group were equivalent to older exercisers who were active at low intensities (Kavanagh, Shephard, Doney, & Pandit, 1973).

Collectively, these studies are consistent with clinical observations that under certain circumstances, behavioral traits and emotional states may influence performance and cardiovascular responses during parts of graded exercise testing and training (American College of Sports Medicine, 1986). Much more study is required before the prevalence of these relationships and their clinical significance can be determined.

Barriers to Training Adaptations

There are also reasons to believe that behavioral and emotional factors may interact with fitness training in ways that can influence chronic adaptations in resting and submaximal physiological responses. Several potential interactions have importance for risk factors associated with chronic disease. Siscovick et al. (1985) have concluded that habitual physical activity is associated with an overall reduction in risk for coronary heart disease, and that studies suggest physical activity may help prevent or control hypertension and diabetes mellitus. Research also suggests that chronic exercise can reduce blood levels of cholesterol and triglycerides, and increase the ratio of high-density lipoprotein to total cholesterol (Haskell, 1984). Each of these changes is viewed as health promoting. Yet, in each area, available research is conflicting. Numerous studies show no change with exercise, and there are in fact, few studies that involve randomized comparisons of exercise with convincing control groups in clinical settings. Also, the types, intensities, durations, and frequencies of physical activity that optimize health-related outcomes are not as well understood as they are for fitness responses (e.g., $\dot{V}O_2$ max).

Because fitness training has not yet been shown to reliably produce a main effect on health risk factors, it may be informative to examine behavioral and emotional characteristics and events that could accompany or interact with the metabolic demands of exercise to produce chronic outcomes. Although exercise studies of these factors are very sparse, there is considerable evidence from behavioral medicine to suggest that psychological interactions can indeed have clinical significance.

Hypertension

The most accepted and plausible explanations for an antihypertensive effect of fitness training are (a) vasodilatory response in peripheral vessels, (b) body fat reduction, (c) regulatory adjustments of diet or metabolism, (d) regulated fluid and sodium excretion rates, and (e) changes in secretion or uptake of catecholamines and renin (Martin & Dubbert, 1985b). In a careful review, Tipton (1984) concluded that most studies show a chronic reduction of 5-25 mmHg in systolic and 3-15 mm Hg in diastolic pressures accompanying exercise training. He further noted that central and peripheral changes in the sympathetic nervous system and in metabolic and kidney functions associated with sodium retention appear to be the most likely mechanisms for these reductions. To specify the main and interactive effects that exercise training exerts on blood pressures, however, Tipton recommended that future studies simultaneously monitor and compare caloric and salt intake, energy expenditure, and behavior modification before, during, and after experimental trials.

Surprisingly, very few studies have examined how psychological stress might be interacting with the metabolic stress of exercise to affect acute or chronic blood pressure responses at rest and during submaximal exertion. A recent review of psychosomatic aspects of essential hypertension discussed the possible impacts of personality, psychotherapy, and exercise independently, but did not discuss their interactions (Taylor & Fortmann, 1983). Because mental stress during submaximal acute exercise can produce transient elevations in systolic blood pressure (Dishman, 1985) whereas relaxation training can acutely and chronically lower resting and submaximal systolic pressures (Gervino & Veazey, 1984; Lobitz, Brammell, & Stoll, 1983), it is perplexing that more exercise training studies have not examined these interactions.

This lack of exercise research is highlighted by results from other treatment approaches suggesting that psychological factors can indeed influence chronic blood pressure outcomes. For example, among borderline hypertensives treated with biofeedback and cognitive restructuring behavior modification, those with resistive hypertension across an 8-week treatment have reported higher levels of psychological distress and more life events than patients whose hypertension was controlled (Egan, Kogan, Garber, & Jarrett, 1983). Our recent 10-week training study (Kiningham, Holly, Sassenrath, Polidora, & Dishman, 1986) showed that changes in rate-pressure product (RPP) at standard submaximal exercise was predicted by changes in $\dot{V}O_2$ max and in self-reported anxiety levels. In 10 of 28 normotensive adults, the relationship between RPP change and fitness change was random; for them changes in anxiety and Type A behavior during the training study mediated the impact fitness changes had on RPP adaptations. We are currently attempting to replicate these results with medicated and unmedicated hypertensive adults. Because anger traits, states, and expression styles have been associated with hypertension and hypertensive responses in both correlational (Spielberger, Jacobs, Russell, & Crane, 1983) and experimental (Steptoe, Melville, & Ross, 1984) studies, we are also examining interactions between training and anger responses.

Hyperlipidemia

Although genetic disposition, gender, age, body fat, fat and carbohydrate consumption, alcohol, smoking, and medication each can influence the composition of plasma lipids and lipoproteins, there is a growing literature showing exercise also exerts an independent influence (Haskell, 1984). Haskell has concluded that reduction of plasma triglyceride levels with exercise is principally an acute response, whereas cholesterol changes appear more chronic. Decreases in very-low-density lipoproteins can also represent a chronic exercise response.

Although the most significant lipemic outcome of exercise training is an elevation in high-density lipoprotein, it is also less reliable, particularly in previously sedentary women. Changes in plasma lipids with exercise conditioning can apparently be influenced by initial lipid levels, body composition, dietary habits, training states, and training volume. As Haskell (1984) has noted, however, neither the interactions of these influences nor the biological mechanisms of exercise effects are understood.

Exercise training studies have, for the most part, ignored the influence of behavioral and emotional responses on plasma lipid responses to acute and chronic exercise. In a recent review of 60 studies published between

1950 and 1982 (mostly in the 1950s and 1960s), Dimsdale and Herd (1982) concluded that plasma lipids are markedly influenced by acute emotional stress. Across a wide range of life events and laboratory stress, substantial changes were reported. Free fatty acids were elevated (8-300%) in 29 of 35 studies; cholesterol was increased (9-36%) in 28 of 43 studies, with no change in 11 studies; and 14 studies of triglyceride change showed equivalent increases, decreases, and no change. The authors of the review duly noted that the available literature in this area is old and has weaknesses. The methods and assays are now dated (e.g., cholesterol was not fractionated, catecholamines were not simultaneously measured, measures were not repeated to determine a subject's characteristic profile within multiple exposures or across stressors, and results may have been influenced by diet). However, other researchers who recently conducted an independent review of an essentially different literature have similarly concluded that "stress, mood, and personality influence lipid metabolism. Differences between individuals in serum cholesterol level, other measures of lipid metabolism, and associated CHD risk seem only partly due to diet" (Van Doornen & Orlebeke, 1982, p. 28). In a review of several behavioral approaches to treating hyperlipidemia, Carmody, Fey, Pierce, Connor, and Matarazzo (1982) suggested that in addition to the interactive effects on lipid changes of dietary and drug regimens, those of exercise, smoking, and Type A behavior should be studied to examine treatment effectiveness and also treatment compliance. This presents a seemingly important challenge for behavioral fitness research.

Blood Platelet Changes

Blood platelet aggregation is believed to contribute to vessel occlusion and thus precipitate infarction of muscle and brain tissue. Because study generally reveals a relationship between stress emotions and in vitro platelet aggregation (Arkel et al., 1982) whereas exercise tends to reduce anxiety and depression (Dishman, 1985), the interaction of exercise training, stress emotions, and platelet physiology is of potential importance for health-related physical fitness. Few studies are available, however, despite early research suggesting a salubrious effect of acute exercise for some types of individuals. In a series of studies (Jenkins et al., 1975) in vitro aggregation reactivity to epinephrine and norepinephrine was tested at rest and following submaximal treadmill exercise (85% max METs). In one trial, an inverse relationship between trait anxiety and duration of aggregation was found at rest; anxious subjects had the shortest aggregation time at rest. After exercise, however, the high anxious showed the greatest increase in aggregation duration. Similarly, in an earlier trial, platelet aggregation after exercise was reduced in Type B subjects, but no change was seen for Type A subjects.

Although the reproducibility of the findings is uncertain, and the clinical significance of in vitro platelet physiology is not confirmed, these early findings were intriguing for several reasons. Plasma levels of norepinephrine rise in response to both metabolic and psychogenic stress (Kohn, Sleet, Carson, & Gray, 1983) and are less responsive to standard exercise intensity after training. Study also suggests that platelet reactivity is influenced by fitness level (Jenkins et al., 1975).

Immune Function

Immunology is an equally intriguing and poorly understood area of possible interaction among fitness training, psychological stress, and health-related adaptations. Kasl (1984) has stated, "Conclusions such as that coping style of emotional suppression is related to lower levels of natural killer cell activity, which in turn leads to a more rapid progression of the disease, are better seen as working hypotheses than as definitive conclusions" (p. 330). Nonetheless, compelling cross-sectional study (McClelland, Floor, Davidson, & Saron, 1980) has shown consistent relationships between low levels of salivary immunoglobulin A and high epinephrine excretion rates among college males who report higher than expected frequency and severity of illness and who also show a personality pattern of inhibited and stressed power motivation. Conversely, other studies suggest that fitness training and level can mediate the impact that stress-coping styles and behavior patterns exert on illness and physiological reactivity to mental stress (Kobasa, Maddi, & Puccetti, 1982; Lake, Suarez, Schneiderman, & Tocci, 1985).

Simon (1984) reviewed 10 studies of the effects of acute exertion (or cross-sectional comparisons of trained and untrained subjects) on various immune function indicators. In general, exercise was associated with a transient increase in granulocytes and lymphocytes (predominantly T-cells), while immunoglobulin levels were unchanged. Most exercise immunology studies have not used control subjects and have not examined exercise training. A recent controlled study by Watson and colleagues (Watson, Moriguchi, Jackson, Werner, & Wilmore, 1986), however, demonstrated decreased killer cell lysis of target cells, increased T-cell mitogenesis and increased mature T-lymphocytes to total lymphocytes ratio following 15 weeks of running 45-60 min per day, 5 days per week at 70-85% of $\dot{V}O_2$ max.

Berk, Tan, Nieman, & Eby (1985) reported a decrease in the ratio of T-lymphocyte helper and suppressor cells (H/S) after graded treadmill exercise to exhaustion; this was independent of fitness and training status. Based on these studies, future research on fitness training and immune function should quantify both stress emotions/behaviors and exercise volume.

Summary

Study of the possible mediating influences of life events, personality, and stress emotions on health-related outcomes of physical fitness and exercise seems particularly timely. The failure of recent clinical trials (Shekelle et al., 1985; U.S. Department of Health and Human Services, 1985; Williams, 1984) to confirm the validity of the encompassing construct of Type A behavior as a predictor of coronary morbidity and mortality, has refocused attention on specific cultural and psychophysiological processes that may more closely relate behavior to health and disease. Further studies of exercise training in preventive medicine settings and studies of free-living physical activity in the population will likely benefit from considering psychological and behavioral variables in areas where metabolic adaptations of exercise offer incomplete explanations for several health-related correlates of physical fitness, physical activity, and exercise training.

References

American College of Sports Medicine. (1986). *Guidelines for graded exercise testing and exercise prescription* (2nd ed.). Philadelphia: Lea & Febiger.

American College of Sports Medicine. (1978). The recommended quantity and quality of exercise for developing and maintaining fitness in healthy adults. *Medicine and Science in Sports and Exercise, 10*(3), vii-ix.

Arkel, Y.S., Haft, J., Buxton, M., Shephard, H., Burghardt, C., & Williams, R. (1982). Emotional arousal and platelet physiology: A review and some original contributions. *Journal of Human Stress, 8*(1), 19-27.

Balke, B. (1974). Prescribing physical activity. In A. Ryan & F. Allman (Eds.), *Sports medicine*. New York: Academic Press.

Barefoot, J.C., Dahlstrom, W.G., & Williams, R.B. (1983). Hostility, CHD incidence, and total mortality: A 25-year follow-up study of 255 physicians. *Psychosomatic Medicine, 45*, 59-63.

Benson, H., Dryer, T., & Hartley, C.H. (1978). Decreased VO_2 consumption during exercise after elicitation of the relaxation response. *Journal of Human Stress, 4*, 38-46.

Berk, L.S., Tan, S.A., Nieman, D.C., & Eby, W.C. (1985). The suppressive effect of stress from acute exhaustive exercise on T lymphocyte helper/ suppressor all ratio in athletes and non-athletes. *Medicine and Science in Sports and Exercise, 17*, 492.

Berman, R., Simonson, E., & Heron, W. (1954). Electrocardiographic effects associated with hypnotic suggestion in normal and coronary sclerotic individuals. *Journal of Applied Physiology, 7*, 89-95.

Blair, S.N., Cooper, K.H., & Gibbons, L.W. (1983). Changes in coronary heart disease risk factors associated with increased treadmill time in 753 men. *American Journal of Epidemiology*, **118**, 352-359.

Blumenthal, J.A., Williams, R.S., Williams, R.B., & Wallace, A.G. (1980). Effects of exercise on the Type A (coronary prone) behavior pattern. *Psychosomatic Medicine*, **42**, 289-296.

Borg, G. (1973). Perceived exertion: A note on "history" and methods. *Medicine and Science in Sports and Exercise*, **5**, 90-93.

Borg, G. (1962). Physical performance and perceived exertion. In *Studia psychologia et paedogogica* (Vol. 11, pp. 1-64). Lund, Sweden: Gleerup.

Bruce, R.A., DeRoven, T.A., & Hossack, K.F. (1980). Value of maximal exercise tests in risk assessment of primary coronary heart disease events in healthy men: Five years' experience of the Seattle Heart Watch Study. *American Journal of Cardiology*, **46**, 371-378.

Burke, E.J., & Collins, M.L. (1984). Using perceived exertion for the prescription of exercise in healthy adults. In R.C. Cantu (Ed.), *Clinical sports medicine* (pp. 93-105). Lexington, MA: Collamore Press.

Canada Fitness Survey: Fitness and lifestyle in Canada. (1983). Ottawa, Canada.

Carmody, T.P., Fey, S.G., Pierce, D.K., Connor, W.E., & Matarazzo, J.D. (1982). Behavioral treatment of hyperlipidemia: Techniques, results, and future directions. *Journal of Behavioral Medicine*, **5**, 91-116.

Carver, C.S., Coleman, E., & Glass, D.C. (1976). The coronary-prone behavior pattern and the suppression of fatigue on a treadmill test. *Journal of Personality and Social Psychology*, **33**, 460-466.

Caspersen, C.J., Powell, K.E., & Christenson, G.M. (1985). Physical activity, exercise, and physical fitness: Definitions and distinctions for health-related research. *Public Health Reports*, **100**, 126-130.

Castell, P.J., & Bluementhal, J.A. (1984). Treadmill performance and reactions to pain of Type A and Type B adults (abstract). *Behavioral Medicine Update*, **6**(2), 14.

Centers for Disease Control. (1985). Status of the 1990 physical fitness and exercise objectives. *Morbidity and Mortality Weekly Report* (U.S. Department of Health and Human Services), **34**, 521-524, 529-531.

Chow, R.J., & Wilmore, J.H. (1984). The regulation of exercise intensity by ratings of perceived exertion. *Journal of Cardiac Rehabilitation*, **4**, 382-387.

Cooper, K.H., Pollock, M.L., Martin, R.P., White, S.R., Linnerud, A.C., & Jackson, A. (1976). Physical fitness levels vs. selected coronary risk factors. *Journal of the American Medical Association*, **236**, 166-169.

Davis, H.A., Gass, G.C., & Bassett, J.R. (1981). Serum cortisol response to incremental work in experienced naive subjects. *Psychosomatic Medicine*, **43**, 127-132.

Denolin, H. (Ed.). (1982). Psychological problems before and after myocardial infarction. *Advances in Cardiology, 19.*

Dimsdale, J.E., & Herd, J.A. (1982). Variability of plasma lipids in response to emotional arousal. *Psychosomatic Medicine, 44,* 413-430.

Dishman, R.K. (Ed.). (1988). *Exercise adherence: Its impact on public health.* Champaign, IL: Human Kinetics.

Dishman, R.K., Patton, R., Smith, J., Weinberg, R., & Jackson, A. (1987). Using perceived exertion to prescribe and monitor exercise training heart rate. *International Journal of Sports Medicine, 8,* 208-213.

Dishman, R.K. (1985). Medical psychology in exercise and sport. *Medical Clinics of North America, 69,* 123-143.

Dishman, R.K., & Gettman, L.R. (1980). Psychobiologic influences on exercise adherence. *Journal of Sport Psychology, 2,* 295-310.

Dishman, R.K., Holly, R.G., & Schelegle, E. (1985). Psychometric, perceptual, and metabolic predictors of self-limited maximal and submaximal treadmill performance (abstract). *Medicine and Science in Sports and Exercise, 17,* 198-199.

Dishman, R.K., Sallis, J., & Orenstein, D. (1985). The determinants of physical activity and exercise. *Public Health Reports, 100,* 158-171.

Dwyer, J., & Bybee, R. (1983). Heart rate indices of the anaerobic threshold. *Medicine and Science in Sports and Exercise, 15,* 72-76.

Egan, K.J., Kogan, H.N., Garber, A., & Jarrett, M. (1983). The impact of psychological distress on the control of hypertension. *Journal of Human Stress, 9*(4), 4-10.

Epstein, L.H. (1984). The direct effects of compliance on health outcome. *Health Psychology, 3,* 385-393.

Epstein, L.H., Wing, R.R., Koeske, R., Ossip, D., & Beck, S. (1982). A comparison of lifestyle change and programmed exercise on weight and fitness changes in obese children. *Behavior Therapy, 13,* 651-665.

Farrell, P.A., Gates, W.K., Maksud, M.G., & Morgan, W.P. (1982). Increases in plasma B-endorphin/B-lipotropin immunoreactivity after treadmill running in humans. *Journal of Applied Physiology: Respiratory, Environmental, and Exercise Physiology, 52,* 1245-1246.

Fielding, J.E. (1982). Effectiveness of employee health improvement programs. *Journal of Occupational Medicine, 24,* 907-916.

Freeman, A.M., Cohen-Cole, S., Fleece, L., et al. (1984). Psychiatric symptoms, Type A behavior, and arrhythmias following coronary bypass. *Psychosomatic Medicine, 25,* 586-589.

George Gallup Organization. (1984). American Health Magazine Survey, New York, NY.

Gervino, E.V., & Veazey, A.E. (1984). The physiologic effects of Benson's Relaxation Response during submaximal aerobic exercise. *Journal of Cardiac Rehabilitation, 4,* 254-261.

Gibbons, L.W., Blair, S.N., Cooper, K.H., & Smith, M. (1983). Association between coronary heart disease risk factors and physical fitness in healthy adult women. *Circulation, 67*, 977-983.

Gillilan, R.E., Chopra, A.K., Keleman, M.H., Stewart, K.J., Ewart, C.K., Keleman, M.D., Valenti, S.A., & Manley, J.D. (1984). Prediction of compliance to target heart rate during walk-jog exercise in cardiac patients by a self-efficacy scale. *Medicine and Science in Sports and Exercise, 16*(2), 115.

Godin, G., Shephard, R.J., & Colantonio, A. (1986). The cognitive profile of those who intend to exercise but do not. *Public Health Reports.*

Goldstein, D.S., Ross, R.S., & Brady, J.V. (1977). Biofeedback heart rate training during exercise. *Biofeedback and Self-Regulation, 2*, 107-126.

Hanson, P. (1984). Clinical exercise testing. In R. Strauss (Ed.), *Sports medicine* (pp. 13-40). Philadelphia: Saunders.

Haskell, W.L. (1984). The influence of exercise on the concentration of triglyceride and cholesterol in human plasma. *Exercise and Sport Sciences Reviews, 12*, 205-244.

Haskell, W.L., Montoye, H.J., & Orenstein, D. (1985). Physical activity and exercise to achieve health-related physical fitness components. *Public Health Reports, 100*, 202-212.

Herd, J.A. (1984). Cardiovascular response to stress in man. *Annual Review of Physiology, 46*, 177-185.

Hockman, C.H., Mauck, H., & Hoff, E.C. (1966). ECG changes resulting from cerebral stimulation: II. A spectrum of ventricular arrhythmias of sympathetic origin. *American Heart Journal, 71*, 695-700.

Hughes, J.R., Crow, R.S., Jacobs, D.R., Mittlemark, M.B., & Leon, A.S. (1985). Physical activity, smoking, and exercise-induced fatigue. *Journal of Behavioral Medicine, 7*, 217-230.

Jenkins, C.D., Stanton, B.A., & Klein, M.D. (1983). Correlates of angina pectoris among men awaiting coronary bypass surgery. *Psychosomatic Medicine, 45*, 141-153.

Jenkins, D., Thomas, G., Olewine, D., Zyzanski, S.J., Simpson, M.T., & Hames, C.G. (1975). Blood platelet aggregation and personality traits. *Journal of Human Stress, 1*(4), 34-46.

Kasl, S.V. (1984). Stress and health. *Annual Review of Public Health, 4*, 319-341.

Kavanagh, T., Shephard, R.J., Pandit, V., & Doney, H. (1970). Exercise and hypnotherapy in the rehabilitation of the coronary patient. *Archives of Physical Medicine and Rehabilitation, 51*, 578-587.

Kavanagh, T., Shephard, R.J., Doney, H., & Pandit, V. (1973). Intensive exercise in coronary rehabilitation. *Medicine and Science in Sports and Exercise, 5*, 34-39.

Kellerman, J.J. (Ed.). (1982). Comprehensive cardiac rehabilitation. *Advances in Cardiology, 31*.

Kiningham, R., Holly, R., Sassenrath, E., Polidora, J., & Dishman, R.K. (1986). Change in rate pressure product after training is predicted by psychometric and metabolic measures (abstract). *Medicine and Science in Sports and Exercise*, **18**(2), S72.

Kittel, F., Kornitzer, M., DeBacker, G., Dramaix, M., Sobolski, J., Oegre, S., & Denolin, H. (1983). Type A in relation to job stress, social and bioclinical variables: The Belgian physical fitness study. *Journal of Human Stress*, **9**(4), 37-45.

Kobasa, S.C., Maddi, S., & Puccetti, M.C. (1982). Personality and exercise as buffers in the stress-illness relationship. *Journal of Behavioral Medicine*, **5**, 391-404.

Kohn, L.M., Sleet, D.A., Carson, J.C., & Gray, R.T. (1983). Life changes and urinary norepinephrine in myocardial infarction. *Journal of Human Stress*, **9**(2), 38-45.

Lake, B.W., Suarez, E.C., Schneiderman, N., & Tocci, N. (1985). The Type A behavior pattern, physical fitness, and psychophysiological reactivity. *Health Psychology*, **4**, 169-187.

Langer, A.W., Obrist, P.A., & McCubbin, J.A. (1979). Hemodynamic and metabolic adjustments during exercise and shock avoidance in dogs. *American Journal of Physiology*, **236**, H225-230.

Levy, A.G. (1914). The genesis of ventricular extrasystoles under chloroform: With special reference to consecutive ventricular fibrillation. *Heart*, **5**, 299-334.

Lo, C.R., & Johnston, D.W. (1984). Cardiovascular feedback during dynamic exercise. *Psychophysiology*, **21**, 199-206.

Lobitz, W.C., Brammell, H.C., & Stoll, S. (1983). Physical exercise and anxiety management training for cardiac stress management in a nonpatient population. *Journal of Cardiac Rehabilitation*, **3**, 683-688.

Londeree, B., & Moeschberger, M.L. (1982). Effect of age and other factors on maximal heart rate. *Research Quarterly on Exercise and Sport*, **53**, 297-304.

Martin, J.E., & Dubbert, P.M. (1985a). Exercise compliance. *Exercise and Sport Sciences Reviews*, **13**, 137-167.

Martin, J.E., & Dubbert, P.M. (1985b). Exercise in hypertension. *Annals of Behavioral Medicine*, **7**, 13-18.

Martin, J.E., Dubbert, P.M., Katell, A., Thompson, J.K., Raczynski, J.R., Lake, M., Smith, P.O., Webster, J.S., Sikova, T., & Cohen, R.E. (1984). The behavioral control of exercise in sedentary adults: Studies 1 through 6. *Journal of Consulting and Clinical Psychology*, **52**, 795-811.

Mason, J.O., & Powell, K.E. (1985). Physical activity, behavioral epidemiology, and public health. *Public Health Reports*, **100**, 113-115.

McClelland, D.C., Floor, E., Davidson, R.J., & Saron, C. (1980). Stressed power motivation, sympathetic activation, immune function, and illness. *Journal of Human Stress*, **6**, 11-19.

Morgan, W.P. (1985). Psychogenic factors and exercise metabolism: A review. *Medicine and Science in Sports and Exercise, 17, 309-317.*

Morgan, W.P., & Borg, G. (1976). Perception of effort in the prescription of physical activity. In T. Craig (Ed.), *The humanistic and mental health aspects of sports, exercise and recreation* (pp. 126-129). Chicago: American Medical Association.

Noble, B.J., Maresh, C.M., & Ritchey, M. (1981). Comparison of exercise sensations between females and males. In J. Borms, M. Hebbelinck, & A. Venerando (Eds.), *Women and sport* (pp. 175-179). Basel, Switzerland: S. Karger.

Oldridge, N.G. (1982). Compliance and exercise in primary and secondary prevention of coronary heart disease: A review. *Preventive Medicine, 11, 56-70.*

Oldridge, N.B., Donner, A.P., Buck, C.W., Jones, N.L., Andrew, G.A., Parker, J.O., Cunningham, D.A., Kavanagh, J., Rechnitzer, P.A., & Sutton, J.R. (1983). Predictors of dropout from cardiac exercise rehabilitation: Ontario Exercise Heart Collaborative Study. *American Journal of Cardiology, 51, 70-74.*

Oldridge, N.B. (1977, April). What to look for in an exercise leader. *The Physician and Sportsmedicine, 5, 85-88.*

Paffenbarger, R.S., Hyde, R.T., Wing, A.L., & Steinmetz, C.H. (1984). A natural history of athleticism and cardiovascular health. *Journal of the American Medical Association, 252, 491-495.*

Pandolf, K.B. (1983). Perceived exertion. *Exercise and Sport Sciences Reviews, 11, 118-158.*

The Perrier study: Fitness in America. (1979). New York: Perrier-Great Waters of France.

Perski, A., & Engel, B.T. (1980). The role of behavioral conditioning in the cardiovascular adjustment to exercise. *Biofeedback and Self-Regulation, 5, 91-104.*

Pollock, M.L. (1988). Prescribing exercise for fitness and adherence. In R.K. Dishman (Ed.), *Exercise adherence: Its impact on public health.* Champaign, IL: Human Kinetics.

Powell, K.E., & Paffenbarger, R.S. (1985). Summary of the workshop on epidemiologic and public health aspects of physical activity and exercise. *Public Health Reports, 100, 118-125.*

Presidents Council on Physical Fitness and Sports. (1973, May). National adult physical fitness survey. *PCPFS Newsletter* (Special Edition).

Presidents Council on Physical Fitness and Sports. (1978). Sports potential for physical fitness. *Physical Fitness Research Digest, 8(1).*

Purvis, J., & Cureton, K. (1981). Ratings of perceived exertion at the anaerobic threshold. *Ergonomics, 24, 295-300.*

Rechnitzer, P.A., Cunningham, D.A., Andrew, G.M., et al. (1983). Relation of exercise to the recurrence rate of myocardial infarction in men. *American Journal of Cardiology, 51, 65-69.*

Reich, P. (1985). Psychological predisposition to life-threatening arrhythmias. *Annual Review of Medicine, 36,* 397-405.

Rejeski, W.J., Morley, D., & Miller, H.S. (1984). The Jenkins Activity Survey: Exploring its relationship with compliance to exercise prescription and MET gain within a cardiac rehabilitation setting. *Journal of Cardiac Rehabilitation, 4,* 90-94.

Rejeski, W.J., Morley, D., & Miller, H. (1983). Cardiac rehabilitation: Coronary-prone behavior as a moderator of graded exercise test performance. *Journal of Cardiac Rehabilitation, 3,* 339-346.

Ross, M.A., Morgan, W.P., & Leventhal, H. (1978). Perceived exertion in adult males possessing either the Type A or Type B behavior pattern (abstract). *Medicine and Science in Sports and Exercise, 10*(1), 51.

Sallis, J.F., Haskell, W.L., Fortmann, S.P., Vranizan, K.M., Taylor, C.B., & Solomon, D.S. (1986). Predictors of adoption and maintenance of physical activity in a community sample. *Preventive Medicine, 15,* 331-341.

Sanne, H.M. (1973). Exercise tolerance and physical training of nonselected patients after myocardial infarction. *Acta Medica Scandinavica, 551*(Suppl.), 1-124.

Schiffer, F., Hartley, H.H., Schulman, C.L., & Abelmann, W.H. (1976). The quiz electrocardiogram: A new diagnostic and research technique for evaluating the relation between emotional stress and ischemic heart disease. *American Journal of Cardiology, 37,* 41-47.

Schlegel, R.P., Wellwood, J.K., Coops, B.E, Gruchow, W.H., & Sharratt, M.T. (1980). The relationship between perceived challenge and daily symptom reporting in Type A vs. Type B post infarct subjects. *Journal of Behavioral Medicine, 3,* 191-204.

Schwartz, G.E., Weinberger, D., & Singer, J.A. (1981). Cardiovascular differentiation of happiness, sadness, anger and fear following imagery and exercise. *Journal of Psychosomatic Medicine, 43,* 343-360.

Shekelle, R.B., Gale, M., Ostfeld, A.M., & Oglesby, P. (1983). Hostility, risk of coronary heart disease, and mortality. *Psychosomatic Medicine, 45,* 109-114.

Shekelle, R.B., Hulley, S.B., Neaton, J.D., Billings, J.H., Borhani, N.O., Gerace, T.A., Jacobs, D.R., Lasser, N.L., Mittlemark, M.B., & Stamler, J. (1985). The MRFIT behavior pattern study: II. Type A behavior and incidence of coronary heart disease. *American Journal of Epidemiology, 122,* 559-570.

Shephard, R.J. (1988). Exercise adherence in corporate settings—personal traits and program barriers. In R.K. Dishman (Ed.), *Exercise adherence: Its impact on public health.* Champaign, IL: Human Kinetics.

Shephard, R.J., Corey, P., & Kavanagh, T. (1981). Exercise compliance and the prevention of a recurrence of myocardial infarction. *Medicine and Science in Sports and Exercise, 13,* 1-5.

Sidney, K., & Shephard, R.J. (1976). Attitude toward health and physical activity in the elderly: Effects of a physical training program. *Medicine and Science in Sports and Exercise*, **8**, 246-252.

Sime, W.E., Buell, J.C., & Eliot, R.S. (1980). Cardiovascular responses to emotional stress (quiz interview) in post-myocardial infarction patients and matched control subjects. *Journal of Human Stress*, **6**, 39-46.

Simon, H.B. (1984). The immunology of exercise: A brief review. *Journal of the American Medical Association*, **16**, 2735-2738.

Siscovick, D.S., LaPorte, R.E., & Newman, J.M. (1985). The disease-specific benefits and risks of physical activity and exercise. *Public Health Reports*, **100**, 180-188.

Smutok, M.A., Skrinar, G.S., & Pandolf, K.B. (1980). Exercise intensity: Subjective regulation by perceived exertion. *Archives of Physical Medicine and Rehabilitation*, **61**, 569-574.

Spielberger, C.D., Jacobs, G., Russell, S., & Crane, R.S. (1983). Assessment of anger: The State-Trait Anger Scale. In J.N. Butcher & C.D. Spielberger (Eds.), *Advances in Personality Assessment* (p. 2).

Steptoe, A., Melville, D., é Ross, A. (1984). Behavioral response demands, cardiovascular reactivity, and essential hypertension. *Psychosomatic Medicine*, **46**, 33-48.

Taylor, C.B., & Fortmann, S.P. (1983). Essential hypertension. *Psychosomatics*, **24**, 433-448.

Thompson, C.E., & Wankel, C.M. (1980). The effects of perceived activity choice upon frequency of exercise behavior. *Journal of Applied Social Psychology*, **10**, 436-444.

Tipton, C.M. (1984). Exercise, training, and hypertension. *Exercise and Sport Sciences Reviews*, **12**, 245-306.

U.S. Department of Health and Human Services. (1985, March). *Measuring psychosocial variables in epidemiologic studies of cardiovascular disease* (NIH Publication No. 85-2270).

van Doornen, L.J.P., & Orlebeke, K.F. (1982). Stress, personality, and serum-cholesterol. *Journal of Human Stress*, **8**, 24-29.

Van Egeren, L.F., Abelson, J.L., & Sniderman, L.D. (1983). Interpersonal and electrocardiographic responses of Type A's and Type B's in competitive socioeconomic games. *Journal of Psychosomatic Medicine*, **27**, 53-59.

Verrier, R.L., & Lown, B. (1984). Behavioral stress and cardiac arrhythmias. *Annual Review of Physiology*, **46**, 155-176.

Watson, R.R., Moriguchi, S., Jackson, J.C., Werner, L., & Wilmore, J.H. (1986). Modification of cellular immune functions in humans by endurance exercise training during B-adrenergic blockade. *Medicine and Science in Sports and Exercise*, **18**, 95-100.

Williams, R.B. (1984). Type A behavior and coronary heart disease. *Behavioral Medicine Update*, **6**(3), 29-35.

Wilson, P.K. (1977). Applications for exercise testing in diagnosis; sports-medicine; and prevention, intervention and rehabilitation exercise programs. In W.E. James & E.A. Amsterdam (Eds.), *Coronary heart disease* (pp. 63-80). Miami, FL: Symposia Specialists Medical Books.

Chapter 5

Prescription for Exercise Adherence

Rod K. Dishman

The problem of dropping out, or noncompliance, in supervised exercise programs has been recognized for many years in cardiac rehabilitation (Oldridge, 1982) and adult fitness (Morgan, 1977). With the recent growth of corporate fitness, similar problems of low rates for adoption and regular participation in the typical worksite program have also been noted (Cox, 1984; Fielding, 1982). Largely through the sustained efforts of several North American researchers, we have begun to understand more who is, and who is not, likely to participate in supervised programs; and we have begun to see some of the reasons why. In fact, our research is beginning to support some of the subjective impressions formed earlier by those who direct clinical programs (see Figure 1). My purpose in this chapter is to review much of this research so that the extent of the problem and an accurate picture of what contributes to it will be illustrated. However, because this has been done several times before by others (Martin & Dubbert, 1982) and myself (Dishman, 1982), my overall goal will be to develop a broader perspective of the exercise compliance issue than has typified past reviews. Several factors support the use of a broader view.

Paradigmatic Issues

First, research on exercise compliance has been spurred largely by practical concerns of service delivery, that is, recruiting and keeping participants in a program. This is pragmatically important, but it has fostered *product* studies (correlating factors in compliance or dropping out) that merely describe programs, participants, and dropouts at single points in time. Very few experimental *process* studies (asking *why* people comply or drop out, and what can be changed) have been attempted. The ones

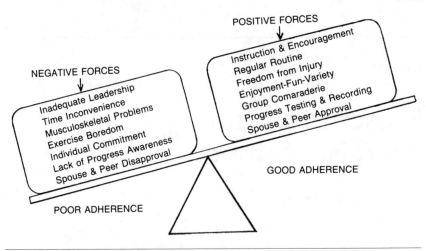

Figure 1 Clinical observations of forces on behavior in adult fitness. *Note.* From "Motivating and Educating Adults to Exercise: Practical Suggestions to Increase Interest and Enthusiasm" by B. Franklin, 1978, *Journal of Physical Education and Recreation*, **49**, p. 13. Copyright 1978 by American Alliance for Health, Physical Education, Recreation, and Dance. Reprinted by permission.

completed have, for the most part, applied general principles of behavior change to exercise settings, but they have not grown out of what is known about exercise programs. There have hardly been any resulting theories about the determinants of exercise compliance. This ultimately limits the generalizability of results from one setting to another. Because many studies that find measurable influences on exercise behavior in groups are not replicated, their actual practical meaning is further limited or remains unknown.

Second, it has become increasingly clear that several factors influencing program participation exert their influence outside the program setting (see Table 1). Thus, viewing exercise behavior only from the narrow perspective of the organized environment is likely to yield disappointing results. For example, changing a program component (e.g., time or convenience) may be inconsequential if barriers to participation originating outside the program remain (e.g., an unsupportive spouse or a busy work schedule).

Third, research increasingly points to the health benefits of multiple-factor behavior interventions. Just as health-risk factors seem to exert their influence in unison, intervention programs that attempt to change more than one behavior may be more effective. Moreover, it has often been assumed that change is easier to accomplish if only one behavior is targeted at a time; more recent thinking, though, suggests that exercise programs that work in a complementary way with other behavior change programs stand not only to yield more healthful outcomes, but may even

Table 1   Factors Associated With Dropout From Exercise Rehabilitation After Myocardial Infarction

Reasons for Dropout	Characteristics of Dropouts
Program type (individualized or group)	Smoker
	Blue-collar occupation
Program problems (staff, facilities)	Overweight
Lack of spousal support	Low self-motivation
Lack of interest, motivation	Angina
Job-related reasons	Physical inactivity
Inconvenience	
Medical and other reasons	

Note. From "Compliance and Dropout in Cardiac Exercise Rehabilitation" by N.B. Oldridge, 1984, *Journal of Cardiac Rehabilitation,* **5,** p. 168. Copyright 1984 by Le Jacq Publishing Company. Reprinted with permission.

promote compliance better, because some behaviors may bolster others. Finally, it remains to be documented who most benefits from supervised exercise programs, personal programs outside the supervised setting, and health alternatives that place less emphasis on fitness-related exercise and more on low-to-moderate intensity physical activity or other stress-coping behaviors.

Methodologic Issues

In examining the existing literature on exercise adherence, it quickly becomes apparent that definitions of exercise behavior vary greatly from study to study. Compliance and adherence are often used interchangeably, even though subjects may be physician-referred or self-referred. There have been no standards for quantifying participation, which might be defined in daily attendance, activity volume, or metabolic change, depending on the study. A dropout from a 6-month study could be an adherent in another that extended just 10 weeks. Because it has been shown that different factors relate to different behaviors at different times (Dishman, 1982; Ward & Morgan, 1984), these definitional issues become very important. Also, a person might leave one program for another, become active again after repeated sedentary relapses, or choose to exercise alone. For all these reasons and more, there appear to be advantages to viewing the problem of ensuring participation in exercise programs as one that extends beyond the staff and facilities of the supervised settings where they occur.

Each of the arguments outlined suggests strongly that more ultimately can be learned and managed about compliance with exercise programs if exercise behavior is viewed from a broad public health perspective, rather than in isolation. This is the overriding goal of this chapter. While previous papers on this topic have suggested practical prescriptions for exercise adherence based on clinical experience (Franklin, 1978; Oldridge, 1977), it is my impression that a continued search for scientifically verifiable determinants of exercise behavior may require a reexamination of how we define exercise adherence and how we ask our questions. The basic assumption of the approach I will take is that we really cannot expect to understand and control exercise participation in preventive medicine settings if we don't understand it outside them, too.

The Scope of the Problem

The importance of understanding exercise adherence has dimensions of both service delivery and the scientific evaluation of exercise outcomes. Controlled exercise trials (10 weeks to 4 years) commonly experience subject attrition rates of 30-70% before study completion (Dishman, 1981b; Morgan, 1977). If dropouts are included in analyses, outcome magnitudes are artificially diluted. If they are excluded, results generalize only to those completing the trial. Even among those who adhere, compliance with the prescribed intensity, duration, and frequency of activity commonly varies between 50-80% (Epstein, Koeske, & Wing, 1984; Martin et al., 1984; Rejeski, Morley, & Miller, 1984). This further mitigates outcome generalizability, because compliance can directly affect health and fitness outcomes (Rejeski et al., 1984; Shephard, Corey, & Kavanaugh, 1981). Thus, the population effectiveness of exercise has not been determined in precise terms, due to behavioral selection biases. Behavioral selectivity also precludes the delivery of exercise and activity outcomes to many whose health might benefit.

Adherence Patterns

Although a few clinical exercise programs report adherence rates of 85-90%, they typically involve small groups (10-40 members), whereas larger (100 or more members), more diverse samples, with greater potential for population representation, commonly experience a 45-55% dropout within 3-6 months (Dishman, 1982; Oldridge, 1982). Among apparently healthy groups who seek out community and commercial exercise settings, dropout rates routinely exceed 50% before a minimum biological adaptation period of 4-10 weeks has elapsed (Martin et al., 1984; Wankel, 1984). Moreover, only 15-30% of eligible employees can be expected to use corporate exercise facilities on a weekly basis (Cox, 1984) and only 38-54% of the users will do so two or more times per week (Fielding, 1982). Population surveys reflect a similar pattern, pointing out that during a given year, 41-51% of adults 18-65 years old do not engage in planned exercise of any kind (Harris and Associates, 1979; U.S. National Center for Health Statistics, 1980). Only one-third are active enough to benefit fitness or health, and only 15% expend energy at a level (1,500 kilocalories per week) of known epidemiologic significance (Harris and Associates, 1979; The General Mills American Family Report, 1978-1979). Only 10% of people over 65 are moderately active on a regular basis (Harris and Associates, 1979).

Despite recent estimates (Canada Fitness Study, 1983; Clarke, 1973; Neilson poll, 1983) of 50-150% increase in involvement in activity that develops cardiopulmonary and musculoskeletal fitness, notably among 18- to 34-year-olds of high socioeconomic status and the well-educated, (Harris and Associates, 1979; The General Mills American Family Report, 1978-1979) nationwide participation rates across all types of physical activity have increased only slightly (4-14%) during the past decade (Harris and Associates, 1979; Clarke, 1973). Community studies suggest that those motivated for fitness, but who have difficulty remaining active, are trying more frequently (Martin et al., 1984; Canada Fitness Study, 1983; Fitness Ontario, 1982). Yet, nearly half of able-bodied American and Canadian adults remain inactive in their leisure time (Harris and Associates, 1979; Canada Fitness Study, 1983). This trend is noteworthy for public health because the balance of current epidemiologic evidence supports a health role for regular physical activity, though it is less clear in specifying the necessity of fitness gains (LaPorte et al., 1984).

Moreover, population involvement rates at given points in time can belie true epidemiologic significance if they do not reflect a period of maintained involvement or adherence for individuals. Among the 36% of adult family members who are active several days per week, about 10% report doing less today than in the past year (The General Mills American Family Report, 1978-1979). The same is reported by 27% of sedentary family members; 55% report their activity level has not changed. Only 18% of American adults state they are likely to increase activity within a year, whereas 42% acknowledge they are unlikely to do so (Harris and Associates, 1979). Of the active, one-fourth believe they will increase involvement (The General Mills American Family Report, 1978-1979); this approximates actual changes (Fitness Ontario, 1982). However, similar proportions of adults from all ages (10-20%) are equally likely to do more or less vigorous exercise in the upcoming year (The General Mills American Family Report, 1978-1979). Among the presently inactive, only 11% believe they will become active during the next year, whereas 62% acknowledge they are unlikely to do so (Harris and Associates, 1979).

One-half of those who enter a community exercise program have experienced previous failures at maintaining an activity routine (Martin et al., 1984). Likewise, one-half of previously inactive community members who intend to initiate regular exercise will do so within 9 months, but one-half of this group will subsequently stop (Fitness Ontario, 1982). During the same time, one-half of those initially active will have become sedentary. Thus, it is unclear how enduring a state either being active or sedentary actually is. We seem to know very little about activity patterns across time for an individual.

Exercise Programs and Public Health

Current activity rates are problematic when contrasted with the health promotion and disease prevention agenda established by the United States Department of Health and Human Services (U.S. Department of Health and Human Services Prevention, 1982). Physical activity objectives for the nation call for attaining the following goals by 1990:

- The proportion of children and adolescents ages 10-17 participating regularly in exercise activities with lifetime carryover should exceed 90%.
- The proportion of adults 18-65 participating regularly in vigorous exercise should exceed 60%.
- One-half of adults 65 years or older should engage in appropriate physical activity (e.g., regular walking, swimming, or other aerobic activity).
- More than 25% of companies and institutions with more than 500 employees should offer employer-sponsored fitness programs.

Available estimates suggest these objectives present a distinct challenge to health professionals. My goal is to review behavioral factors shown to be related to habitual physical activity and adherence to exercise programs. This examination can help explain why current activity patterns exist and can specify what must likely be changed to alter them. In the process, populations and target variables will be isolated, which may guide interventions. Although factors that determine initial involvement in physical activity and exercise can differ from determinants of maintained involvement or adherence (Dishman, 1982, 1984b), my principal focus will be on adherence. Some who have no intention of becoming active can likely be persuaded to adopt an activity program, but the likelihood of continued participation may increase or decrease, depending on the number of prior attempts. However, the act of beginning an activity routine has no established epidemiologic significance, and the problem of insuring increased participation does not appear to be exclusively one of fostering initial involvement (Dishman, 1982; Morgan, 1977). Hence, the decision to make long-term behavior the most closely examined dependent variable seems justified.

Behavioral Influences on Exercise Adherence and Physical Activity

The known determinants of physical activity and exercise can be categorized as features of the person, past and present environments, lifestyle habits, activity settings, and activity itself (Dishman, 1982, 1984b). For clarity, these will be presented independently, but only a few have shown promise for behavioral invariance across settings, populations, and time periods. Any one may be influential under certain conditions; they likely interact in complex ways, and their relative importance can change. A conceptual framework is presented in Table 2 to illustrate that exercise determinants can be either psychological, biological, or situational in origin. These groupings are not independent of each other, however. Several examples will illustrate the existence of a complex interaction between them so that the decision to exercise (or not to) is seen to be probably a product of abstract conceptual beliefs (thoughts) and concrete sensory perceptions (feelings) that a person brings to, or experiences during, exercise. These likely interact with situational factors in the exercise setting, some of which may be readily changed. Others are largely environmental characteristics or personal traits that are difficult to alter (Dishman, 1984). Table 2 illustrates this interactive view. The organization of the review that follows is designed to (a) cover in a representative way what is now known, (b) group together findings that share common dimensions either in defining concepts of exercise behavior or variables of practical significance, and (c) suggest concerns for future study and application.

The overall goal here is to give a broad view that can guide future attempts at conceptually based research and empirically based program decisions designed to understand and facilitate exercise behavior. To help accomplish this, the review is divided into seven sections: (a) Personal Activity History; (b) Social History and Physical Activity: Family and Friends; (c) Knowledge, Attitudes, and Beliefs; (d) Other Health Beliefs and Exercise: Attitudes versus Behavior; (e) Barriers to Exercise; (f) Reinforcement for Participation; (g) Characteristics of Those Who Resist Exercise.

Personal Activity History

In clinical exercise programs, past participation in a program is the most reliable predictor of current participation (Dishman, 1982, 1984a; Martin et al., 1984; Morgan, 1977; Oldridge, 1982). The strength of this relationship appears to be a function of time elapsed from the outset of involvement. This holds for men and women alike in programs for adult fitness and for treating coronary heart disease and obesity. The typical dropout

Table 2   Factors Influencing the Decision to Stay With an Exercise Program

The Exerciser	Situational Factors
Biological	*Lifestyle-related*
Traits	Support from "significant others"
Body composition	Vocational status
Aerobic fitness	Recreational activity patterns
Health status (CHD)	Smoking
Asymptomatic vs. diseased	
Multiple heart attacks	*Exercise setting*
	Accessibility or convenience
Psychological	Small group vs. alone
Traits	Moderate intensity
Self-motivation	(e.g., < 85% max HR)
Other "personality" factors	
(extraversion, attitudes/beliefs,	*Behavior change strategies*
coronary-prone behavior)	Contracts
Sensory states	Behavioral contingencies
Symptomatic pain	Social reinforcement
Perceived exertion	Benefit/cost evaluation
	Self-monitoring
	Stimulus-cuing
	Sensory distraction
	Goal setting
	Tailored to the exerciser
	Daily flexibility
	Perceived choice of activity
	Distal vs. proximal (i.e., long-
	term vs. immediate)

Note. From "Motivation and Exercise Adherence" by R.K. Dishman, 1984, in J. Silva and R. Weinberg (Eds.), *Psychological Foundations of Sport*, Champaign, IL: Human Kinetics. Copyright 1984 by John Silva and Robert Weinberg. Reprinted by permission.

rate is graphically described by a negative acceleration line within the initial 3-6 months, which then plateaus and continues a gradual, linear form across the next 12-18 months (see Figure 2).

Individuals who are still active after 6 months are more likely to remain active a year later (Dishman, 1981b). The impact of previous activity outside the clinical setting is less clear. In one walking program for healthy,

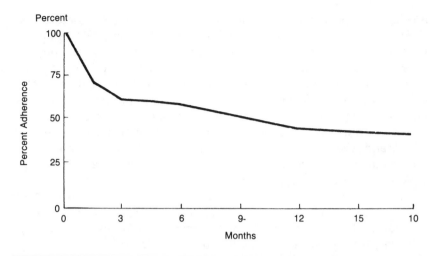

Figure 2 Typical adherence rate in supervised exercise programs. *Note.* From *Essentials of Fitness* by Harold B. Falls, Ann M. Baylor, and Rod K. Dishman, © 1980 by Saunders College–Holt, Rinehart and Winston. Reprinted with permission by Holt, Rinehart and Winston, Inc.

middle-aged women, the amount of routine walking and stair climbing prior to enrollment was associated with walking mileage in the clinical setting (C. Bayles, unpublished observations). A parallel, reliable predictor of dropout from exercise rehabilitation among male post-myocardial infarction patients has been inactive leisure time (Oldridge, 1982). However, self-reported intensity, duration, and frequency of pre-program exercise among males apparently healthy and males at risk for coronary heart disease have not been related to length of stay in a preventive exercise program or to sessions attended per month (Dishman, 1981b).

Although a cross section of active male participants in adult fitness programs is likely to reveal a sport background (Harris, 1970), no prospective relationship has been seen between adherence to clinical exercise programs and participation in interscholastic or intercollegiate athletics (Dishman, 1981b; Morgan, 1977). About two-thirds of all adults with an interscholastic or intercollegiate history in two or more sports are regularly active. They are two to three times as likely as former nonathletes to engage in such strength and endurance exercise as bicycling, calisthenics, jogging, and swimming (Clarke, 1973). Yet, former participants in a single sport and those with no sport history each show a 50% likelihood of regular exercise. By the age of 45, male, former intercollegiate athletes can become even less active in leisure time than former nonathletes (Montoye et al., 1957).

The impact of youth sports on adult exercise patterns is not known (Powell & Dysinger, in press). Although high school sport participation is believed to exert relatively greater influence on adult behavior than does elementary participation (Loy, McPherson, & Kenyon, 1978) empirical study shows that school sport participation is unrelated to adult physical activities (Dishman, in press). Conversely, a positively perceived physical education experience at the elementary school level better predicts adherence to an adult running program than does physical education at post-elementary levels. There appears to be a stronger relationship between youth sport participation and involvement in organized adult sport (Harris and Associates, 1979; Loy et al., 1975; The Miller Lite Report, 1983). This seems particularly true among females (Greendorfer, 1983).

Skill development appears to be a necessary, but not sufficient, behavioral influence, but this can occur outside of school or organized sport environments. It appears to be a more important influence for competitive, rather than recreational, leisure sport, where continuity of the type of activity from adolescence to adulthood is more reliable (Loy et al., 1978; The Miller Lite Report, 1983). Thus, while sport experience can be an agent in socializing adult roles, it seems frequently overridden by other personal and environmental influences that exert a more immediate impact in adulthood. Furthermore, it is difficult to separate behavioral influence learned from sport involvement (e.g., activity skills and interests) from the influence of other personal traits that may mediate both youth sport involvement and adult exercise patterns. For example, personality, body build and composition, and functional tolerance all have been related to both sport success and adult activity patterns (Dishman, 1982, 1984), yet have largely heritable origins.

Organized sport experience can contribute knowledge and skills useful for activity in later years, and former interscholastic and intercollegiate athletes hold more positive attitudes toward physical activity and higher perceptions of physical ability than do former nonathletes (Morgan, 1977; Harris, 1970; The Miller Lite Report, 1983). These attitudes and self-perceptions are related to involvement in middle school and high school sport (Loy et al., 1978) and to leisure sport participation in adulthood (The Miller Lite Report, 1983), but are unrelated to adherence in adult fitness programs or leisure exercise (Andrew et al., 1981; Martin & Dubbert, 1982; Morgan, 1977). It is not known if factors related to dropping out of youth sport (Gould & Horn, 1984) influence adult activity patterns.

Social History and Physical Activity: Family and Friends

Prior to socialization into organized sport, strong normative influences on physical activity are exerted on children by peers (Loy et al., 1978). These are sex-linked through adolescence but can become independent of gender in adulthood. Peer influence increases with age and moves from the neighborhood in childhood to the place of employment by adulthood.

Peers can operate in parallel with organized sport involvement by modeling skills and providing social reinforcement. Like-gender peer models are particularly important for influencing female participation (Greendorfer, 1983). It is not, however, clearly known to what degree peers influence a behavioral change or, conversely, are chosen to match existing interests and skills.

Physical activity patterns of the family exert direct and indirect influences throughout one's life span on participation in organized sport (Greendorfer, 1983), clinical exercise programs (Dishman, 1982; Morgan, 1977; Oldridge, 1982) and leisure physical activity (The General Mills American Family Report, 1978-1979). During one's childhood years, family influence exceeds that of the school by modeling interests and skills, reinforcing behavior, and providing activity environments. This is largely gender-specific. Activity modeling and support by the mother is particularly a strong influence for female participation in sport and exercise during later years (Greendorfer, 1983). It is also likely that heritable interests and abilities also influence activity success and habits. Among children whose parents were interested in athletic participation, 74-80% are regularly active (Harris and Associates, 1979). However, more than half of those whose parents were not active in sports are also active.

Support by a spouse is a consistent influence on adherence to clinical exercise programs, and the attitude toward involvement held by the spouse is more reliably important than that held by the participant (Andrew et al., 1981). Spouse support takes the form of both normative reinforcement and removal of barriers to activity. Among those choosing exercise, only 37% have spouses that share their preference over forms of sedentary leisure.

Among parents who participate in sport, nearly 60% spend one-half of their involvement participating with their family (Harris and Associates, 1979). Throughout the entire population, however, only one-third of adult family members engage in planned exercise several times a week (The General Mills American Family Report, 1978-1979), and this does not differ from nationwide estimates (Harris and Associates, 1979). During leisure time, only one in four American family members prefers to exercise rather than relax at home or with sedentary entertainment outside the home (The General Mills American Family Report, 1978-1979). Among regularly exercising family members, single parents of high socioeconomic status are highly represented as are the age groups 18-34 years and 65 years and over. Among family members, place of residence, gender, and employment status are each equally represented and do not appear to influence exercise (The General Mills American Family Report, 1978-1979). Throughout the entire population urban males are more likely to be active in leisure (Harris and Associates, 1979). Of all family members, 80% feel they presently do not exercise enough (The General Mills American Family Report, 1978-1979).

The principal barriers against increasing activity levels as perceived by family members, include lack of time (43%), lack of willpower (16%), an attitude of "just don't feel like it" (12%), medical problems (9%), and lack of energy (8%). Notably, however, regular exercisers and those who are sedentary do not differ in their perceptions of activity barriers, with the exception that twice as many sedentary (13%) than the active (7%) "just don't feel like it." This similarity challenges the validity of perceived barriers as activity determinants among those who have positive intentions to exercise. Rather, it suggests that inactivity among adult family members is more attributable to insufficient intrinsic reinforcement than to poor attitudes, lack of intention, or perceived barriers. By adulthood, family influence can facilitate participation, but lack of family support is not a major deterrent to activity (The General Mills American Family Report, 1978-1979), nor is it perceived as a facilitator of increased involvement (Harris and Associates, 1979).

Knowledge, Attitudes, and Beliefs

Regular exercisers are likely to have had more years of public education than non-exercisers (Harris and Associates, 1979; The General Mills American Family Report, 1978-1979; Harris, 1970), while participation in recreational sport seems less related to formal education (The Miller Lite Report, 1983). However, there is little relationship between increasing the knowledge, beliefs, or attitudes people hold about exercise, and their increased adherence to an exercise regimen (Dishman, 1982, 1984a; Meyer et al., 1980). This applies to both clinical programs and community activity. The inactive are as likely to view exercise as a positive health behavior as are the active (Harris and Associates, 1979; The General Mills American Family Report, 1978-1979; Andrew et al., 1981). The behavioral importance of attitudes and beliefs is, however, specific in impact. Those who strongly value exercise as a health behavior, believe they have control over health outcomes, and expect health benefits from exercise are more likely to select high-intensity exercise and to engage in higher volumes of it than are those holding weak or negative beliefs (Shephard, 1978; Sonstroem, 1982). Knowledge of health and exercise is associated with regular activity of moderate intensity (e.g., routine walking) for both men and women but does not predict participation in vigorous exercise (Dishman, 1982, 1984a). Inactive members of low socioeconomic groups are relatively uninformed about the health benefits of exercise and its appropriate forms or amounts, (Harris and Associates, 1978; Canada Fitness Study, 1983; Dishman, 1984b), but through the entire population only 4% of the currently inactive and 2% of the active believe more information on fitness benefits would likely increase their participation (Harris and Associates, 1978).

Lack of confidence in the ability to be active or to maintain exercise can reflect past history and can perpetuate inactivity. However, perceived ability does not insure activity (Dishman, 1982) even though self-estimates of likely adherence can be effective prognosticators of actual behavior (Meyer et al., 1980).

Other Health Beliefs and Exercise: Attitudes Versus Behavior

To clarify their true impact, it is useful to view exercise and physical activity within broader health attitudes (The General Mills American Family Report, 1978-1979). Six of ten adult family members report concern over behavioral health. They believe it should not be taken for granted and that actively pursuing a preventive approach is worthwhile. Four of ten are complacent and deal with health problems only on a crisis basis. Those who are concerned are likely to report they have changed personal and family lifestyles, including exercise, to foster health. They reportedly exercise two or three times a week and feel well-informed about health behavior. In fact, perceived changes in lifestyle health behaviors can be the strongest correlate of reported increases in activity levels (Fitness Ontario, 1982). Yet, other evidence notes that health beliefs can be behaviorally incongruent (The General Mills American Family Report, 1978-1979). Even though most adults verbally endorse a preventive lifestyle, 75% paradoxically believe themselves to be in good health as long as they experience no physical symptoms, and 54% deny that a serious illness could befall a member of their family.

Thus, health concern and belief in the benefits of healthy behavior do not alone produce the behavior. Though 80% of family members believe they should exercise more than they currently do, the inactive are as likely to share this view as the regularly active; yet, 27% of the inactive are actually doing less today than a year ago. Further, though many more of those concerned about health report they exercise weekly than do the complacent (43% versus 25%) the majority of both groups are inactive (The General Mills American Family Report, 1978-1979). In contrast, a decade earlier 40% of American adults felt they did not get enough exercise, while the inactive were twice as likely as the active (63% versus 33%) to believe they exercised enough (Clarke, 1973). More recently, one-half of the inactive feel their daily activity is sufficient exercise without participating in sport, but only 15% of the vigorously active share this perspective (Harris and Associates, 1979). However, the increase in awareness of the value of physical activity through the past decade, coupled with a steady proportion of adults who do not exercise at all (41-51%) (Harris and Associates, 1979; U.S. National Health Statistics, 1980), argues against thinking that knowledge and beliefs about exercise benefits are important determinants of actual behavior (Fitness Ontario, 1981).

This view is reinforced by corporate and community research suggesting that knowledge and beliefs of health benefits may motivate initial involvement, but feelings of enjoyment and well-being are stronger reinforcers for continued participation (Shepard. 1978). Six in ten people are aware of physical fitness and exercise promotions (Clarke, 1973), and 36% believe exercise is underemphasized as a health issue (The General Mills American Family Report, 1978-1979). But only 10-17% report that their awareness of exercise promotions has motivated them to be more active (McIntosh, 1980), and it is unknown how many of this group were previously sedentary. Estimates suggest that among regular exercisers, one-fourth have been told to do so by their physician, but only 3% report this is the reason for their activity (Clarke, 1973). This is observed despite the fact that 75% of family members express confidence in their physicians (The General Mills American Family Report, 1978-1979) and substantial proportions of both the inactive (43%) and the active (32%) state that a physician's recommendation would likely increase their involvement in sport (Harris and Associates, 1979).

Thus, while the active are more knowledgeable about fitness and exercise information, it is unclear whether this precipitates or follows their involvement. Available evidence collectively suggests that regular participation is influenced as much by expecting and valuing immediate, concrete, physical and emotional reinforcement, as it is by abstract knowledge and beliefs of future health benefits (Harris and Associates, 1979; Martin & Dubbert, 1982; Lindsay-Reid, & Osborn, 1980). Whether this expectation can be facilitated in the absence of actual experience remains undemonstrated.

In both clinical and community exercise programs, the act of rationally evaluating the anticipated benefits and costs of being active (see Table 3) has consistently facilitated increased participation, or a return to activity among the previously active (Wankel, 1984).

This effect has been demonstrated only for short time periods (4-10 weeks) among the already motivated. As such, it appears to prompt an existing behavioral skill or serve as a reminder of an earlier exercise decision, but it does not show that knowledge of the benefits and risks of physical activity is a singularly important determinant of behavior (Harris and Associates, 1979; Dishman, 1987).

Barriers to Exercise

No evidence supports the idea that the financial cost of physical activity is a barrier to participation (Harris and Associates, 1979). Although members of high socioeconomic groups are more likely to be aware of the importance of fitness and sports and to exercise regularly (Harris and

Table 3   Balance-Sheet Procedure

Systematic exploration between interviewer and participant of anticipated outcomes

Self-disclosing interview in which the participant reports anticipated outcomes to interviewer

Interviewer reinforces positive statements and buffers anticipated negative outcomes

---

Note. From "Decision-Making and Social-Support Strategies for Increasing Exercise Involvement" by L.M. Wankel, 1984, *Journal of Cardiac Rehabilitation,* 4, p. 126. Copyright 1984 by Le Jacq Publishing Company. Reprinted with permission.

Associates, 1979; The General Mills American Family Report, 1978-1979), those of lower socioeconomic groups are equally likely to purchase specialized equipment for recreational sport. Middle income groups are the most likely to anticipate increased sport expenditures during the coming year (Harris and Associates, 1978). Most fitness-related activities remain low-cost, and surveys indicate that enrollment fees are not perceived as barriers to participation in community, corporate, or clinical exercise programs. Only 10% of the public report that less expensive facilities would likely increase sport involvement, while the already active are twice as likely as the inactive (13% versus 6%) to hold this view (Harris and Associates, 1979).

Depositing a fee that is returnable upon successful program completion is a common and effective short-term intervention for facilitating exercise adherence (Dishman, 1982; Martin & Dubbert, 1982), but commercial exercise programs experience dropout rates similar to other programmatic exercise settings (Wankel, 1984), faring only as well as corporate and community programs that provide free access to exercise and activity facilities (Cox, 1984; Fielding, 1982; Martin et al., 1984). Moreover, only 17% of adult family members feel money is a barrier to good health (The General Mills American Family Report, 1978-1979). Perceived need for medical clearance might be an exercise barrier to some, since three of four family members feel that medical checkups cost too much for the average family (The General Mills American Family Report, 1978-1979).

Surveys of habitual runners (Sacks & Sachs, 1981) reveal that only among the most committed (less than 10%) do weather conditions have no impact on activity patterns. Most (50%) commonly interrupt their routines if the environment is inclement, but it is not known how many seek substitute settings. The type of leisure sport participation is influenced by seasonal availability, but most who are active remain involved in activities year-round (Canada Fitness Study, 1983; The Miller Lite Report, 1983). In a like manner, climate clearly influences choices of outdoor leisure activities (The Miller Lite Report, 1983), but it is unknown if overall participation rates differ by region. Highly active (expending 1500 Kcal/wk) American adults are more likely to live in the West and Midwest, while inactive adults live in the East and South (Harris and Associates, 1979). This distribution is as likely to reflect age and socioeconomic factors as climate, however. Although 27% of the public state that nicer weather would likely increase their sport involvement, nearly twice as many active as inactive people (33%-18%) believe this to be the case (Harris and Associates, 1979).

Access to facilities is a necessary, but not sufficient, facilitator of community sport and exercise participation (Harris and Associates, 1979). It is perceived as an important participation influence (Fitness Ontario, 1981), particularly among the elderly (Shephard, 1978). Also, both perceived convenience of the exercise setting and its actual proximity to home or place of employment are consistent discriminators between those who choose to enter or forego involvement, and between those who adhere or dropout, in clinical exercise programs (Andrew et al., 1981; Martin & Dubbert, 1982; Oldridge, 1982). Yet, in one unsupervised exercise program, those most likely to drop out actually lived closer to the chosen activity setting, even though they perceived inconvenience as a factor leading to their return to inactivity (Gettman, Pollock, & Ward, 1983). Also, the already active are twice as likely as the inactive (22% versus 10%) to feel that greater availability of facilities would increase their participation (Harris and Associates, 1979).

A similar incongruity between perceived and actual barriers is seen for the time element, lack of which is the principal and most prevalent reason given for dropping out of clinical and community exercise programs (Dishman, 1982; Gettman et al., 1983; Oldridge, 1982) and for inactive lifestyles (Harris and Associates, 1979; The General Mills American Family Report, 1978-1979; Sacks and Sachs, 1981). For many, however, this apparently reflects equally a lack of interest, intention, or commitment to physical activity, because regular exercisers are as likely as the sedentary to view time as an activity barrier (Harris and Associates, 1979; The General Mills American Family Report 1978-1979). Also, the already active are twice as likely as the now inactive (22% versus 10-11%) to believe a 4-day work week or more flexiblity in the daily work schedule would lead to increased likelihood of sport involvement and fitness (Harris and Associates, 1979). Moreover, among family members, working women are more likely than nonworking women to be regular exercisers, one-half of single parents are regularly active, compared to one-third in other parental groups (The General Mills American Family Report, 1978-1979).

Perceived discomfort during an exercise program of running has precipitated dropping out among women regardless of the actual metabolic strain (% VO_2 max) (Dishman, 1984). However, no difference in cumulative dropout rate has been seen between male post-myocardial infarction patients randomly assigned to either high volume (60-85% $\dot{V}O_2$ max, 4 days/wk) or low volume (50% $\dot{V}O_2$ max, 1 day/wk) activity in a 4-year clinical exercise trial (Oldridge et al., 1983). However, the physically untrained perceive a standard activity intensity as greater than do the trained (Pandolph, 1983). Moreover, the intensity of activity does appear to be a determinant of participation in community leisure exercise (Sallis, Haskell, Fortmann, et al., 1986). While more men than women adopt vigorous exercise, such as running, during a year's time a comparatively higher proportion of women take up such moderate activities as routine walking or stair climbing. Furthermore, moderate activities show a dropout rate roughly one-half of that typically seen for vigorous exercise. Injuries from high-intensity running can directly lead to dropout, but this should not become a problem for the typical case until durations of 45 minutes and frequencies of 5 days per week are performed by the previously untrained (Pollock et al., 1977).

Reinforcement for Participation

Cross-sectional studies and surveys of adults suggest that chronic and acute emotional states influence activity patterns. Regular exercisers consistently show mood profiles more favorable than sedentary cohorts (Harris and Associates, 1978) and are less likely to report a depressive or neurotic personality (Lobstein, Mosbacher, & Ismail, 1983). Also, mood disturbance at entry predicts who will drop out from adult fitness programs for apparently healthy men and women (Blumenthal, Williams, Wallace, Williams, & Needles, 1982; Ward & Morgan, 1984). Moreover, daily somatic complaints are directly related to low metabolic tolerance for exercise (Collingwood et al., 1983). Among patients who presented clinically elevated scores on the Cornell Medical Index of perceived organic and emotional health, only a small proportion eligible for supervised exercise entered a program (Shephard, 1978). Those with higher scores can be expected to select low-intensity, low-frequency activity, independent of their metabolic tolerance for exercise. Among the highly committed and self-regulating, however, symptom management with exercise can be a strong reinforcement for habitual involvement (Sacks & Sachs, 1981) and has even been implicated in excessive dependence on exercise (Morgan, 1979). In addition, long-term exercise goals related to improved health and fitness are more predictive of continued exercise involvement than are short-range expectations (Martin et al., 1984; Harris and Associates, 1978). However, their effectiveness is probably dependent on knowledge of the time course for fitness and health changes and patience for change to occur gradually (Dishman, 1987).

Our measure of self-motivation (Dishman & Ickes, 1981) has consistently predicted length of involvement with exercise programs in community, corporate, and clinical settings (Dishman, 1984b; Fitness Ontario,

Table 4   Psychobiologic Prediction Using Self-Motivation and Body Composition

Attendance	Result	Percent	Base	Gain
Adhere	36 of 41	88%	48%	40%
Dropout	9 of 35	26%	46%	−20%

Note. From "Adherence Patterns of Healthy Men and Women Enrolled in an Adult Exercise Program" by A. Ward and W.P. Morgan, 1984, *Journal of Cardiac Rehabilitation*, **4**, p. 149. Copyright 1984 by Le Jacq Publishing Company. Adapted by permission.

Table 5   Estimating Dropouts in Sentry Insurance Program

All factors	88%
Self-motivation and smoking	82%
Self-motivation	79%

Note. Reprinted from *Corporate Fitness & Recreation*, 2:5, p. 32, 1983, with the permission of the author, William J. Stone, EdD, and Brentwood Publishing Corp, a Prentice-Hall/Simon & Schuster unit of Gulf + Western, Inc.

1982; Ward & Morgan, 1984). These predictions have been aided by the inclusion of body weight and composition into standardized regression and discriminant function equations. To my knowledge, our psychobiologic prediction model is the first screening approach to show some generalizability to independent samples (see Table 4). However, it does not as reliably predict daily participation or dropping out of supervised settings (see Table 5) (Dishman, 1987; Wankel, 1984; Ward & Morgan, 1984). This suggests that self-motivated people may be equally likely to select activity environments that do not rely on professional or social support. They also appear less sensitive to activity barriers, so that inconvenience, lack of social support, the type of activity, competing lifestyle behaviors, or failure to quickly reach a training goal can exert less negative impact on the decision to be active (see Table 6) (Dishman, 1987).

For many, self-motivated physical activity stems from rational goal setting and self-reinforcement of a valued behavior (Dishman & Ickes, 1981). It is believed that many who have the intention to be active but remain sedentary lack these self-regulatory skills; study indicates that interventions incorporating appropriate goal orientations and planning, together with conscientious self-monitoring and self-reward, can support partici-

Table 6   Jackson, Mississippi, Community Exercise Studies Barriers to
Participation

Subject Factors	Program Factors	Consequent Factors	Other Factors
Poor "self-motivation"	Little/no personalized feedback or praise during exercise	Injury	Weather (lower temperatures; precipitation)
	Inflexible program goals	Exercise enjoyment level	Job change/move
	Exercises alone, uses distance goals		Competing activities
	Higher intensity exercise		Vacations/travel
	Somatic preoccupation during exercise		

Note. Barriers to community exercise programs. Courtesy of John Martin, Department of Psychology, San Diego State University, San Diego, California.

pation among the activity-intentioned but undermotivated (Martin et al., 1984). The usefulness of these goal-setting and reinforcement skills for maintaining involvement has as yet been demonstrated only for short periods (4-10 weeks) among those already motivated to adopt activity (see Table 7). A short-term increase in activity of 20% above expected levels can be anticipated (Martin & Dubbert, 1982). This may, however, have longer-term carryover, since self-report evidence supports the view that intrinsically concrete rewarding states (e.g., feeling better or receiving enjoyment from personal mastery) can supplant initial abstract incentives (e.g. anticipation of health benefits, desire for weight loss); these states may reduce reliance on cognitive self-regulation by fostering more reliably motivating sensory reinforcements (Harris and Associates, 1978; Martin & Dubbert, 1982; Sacks & Sachs, 1981).

Even among the active who are well-intentioned and who value benefits from their participation, unexpected disruptions in activity routines or settings can interrupt or conclude previously continuous exercise programs (Dishman, 1984; Oldridge, 1982). Such life occurrences as relocation, medical events, and travel can impede the continuity of activity reinforcement and create new activity barriers. It is believed that they have

Table 7   Components of a Behavioral Contract

A written agreement

Behavior to be changed is clearly described so that it is evident when the behavior occurs

Consequences of the behavior (and perhaps of the absence of the behavior) are clearly specified so that the individual is aware of what will be gained or forfeited by compliance or noncompliance

Criterion for time or frequency limitations should be stated

Note. From "Behavioral Management Strategies for Improving Health and Fitness" by J.E. Martin and P.M. Dubbert, 1984, *Journal of Cardiac Rehabilitation,* p. 202. Copyright 1984 by Le Jacq Publishing Company. Reprinted by permission.

less impact as the activity habit becomes more established (Dishman, 1982); their impact can be diminished also if the individual anticipates and plans their occurrence, recognizes them as only temporary impediments, and develops self-regulatory skills (King & Frederiksen, 1984).

Setting management appears to be a particularly important behavioral skill for those who desire an increase in activity level but have a history of difficulty in achieving one (see Table 8). A daily routine consistently in a convenient place and time, a routine that is flexible enough to accommodate existing activity preferences and daily fluxes in motivation, but is planned to achieve tangible long-term activity objectives within a reasonable time (e.g. 6-10 weeks), should facilitate the reinforcing potential

Table 8   Requirements for Maximizing Initial Participation in Employee Fitness Programs

---

Management support and encouragement

Advisory committee with representatives from all facets of corporate life

Employee involvement in program

Proper promotion of program

Convenience

Conducive environment

Professional leadership

Note. From "Fitness and Lifestyle Programs for Business and Industry: Problems in Recruitment and Retention" by M.H. Cox, 1984, *Journal of Cardiac Rehabilitation,* **4,** p. 138. Copyright 1984 by Le Jacq Publishing Company. Reprinted by permission.

of participation, while minimizing major impediments (Martin et al., 1984). Understanding that relapses are normal and reversible seems important to insuring that attempts to be active are persistent (Marlatt & Gordon, 1980). For many adults, personalized social support from program staff or an activity partner of similar interests and ability are potent exercise and activity reinforcers (Dishman, 1984; Martin et al., 1984; Wankel, 1984). This support can provide an important behavioral boost for those who intend to be active and can be as effective for those who do as for those who do not possess high commitment skills or internalized reinforcement systems (Wankel, 1984).

Characteristics of Those Who Resist Exercise

Smokers and blue-collar workers are likely dropouts from rehabilitative exercise programs for post-myocardial infarction patients (Oldridge, 1982), suggesting that occupational status can parallel socioeconomic and education status in signaling populations at high risk for inactivity. These factors also describe those likely to forego use of corporate exercise facilities (Cox, 1984; Fielding, 1982) and those who are relatively inactive in leisure time (Fitness Ontario, 1981). Their influence, however, appears to be specific to preventive medicine and fitness settings and activities, because neither smoking nor occupational status is related to participation in leisure sport (Harris and Associates, 1978; The Miller Lite Report, 1983).

The overweight also are less likely to stay with a fitness program (Dishman, 1981a), and the obese may better respond to such alternative routines of increased activity as walking or climbing modes (Epstein et al., 1984). Even so, excess weight is still a barrier to activity (Brownell & Stunkard, 1980), and the obese are less responsive to alternative activity forms than are normal weight inactives (Brownell, Stunkard, & Albaum, 1980). Even in gentle walking programs, 60-70% of the obese will stop within 6-12 months (Brownell & Stunkard, 1980; Epstein et al., 1984).

Circulatory disability or low metabolic tolerance (VO_2 max) for physcial activity are not alone reliable predictors of adherence to clinical exercise programs (Martin & Dubbert, 1982; Morgan, 1977); however, among apparently healthy males, initial fitness predicts higher volume of participation in a year-long running program. Males in cardiac rehabilitation exercise programs are more likely to adhere if they have documented heart disease, angina, or have had one myocardial infarction (Dishman, 1981, 1982; Oldridge, 1982). These factors provide concrete signs of health vulnerability and can interact with beliefs about the health benefits of exercise in order to facilitate participation (Dishman, 1982, 1984b).

Neither beliefs, disability, nor health risk factors alone seem sufficient to prompt exercise behavior, however. Males at risk for coronary heart disease are less likely to enter an exercise program (Cox, 1984) or adhere after entry (Oldridge, 1982; Shephard & Cox, 1980). Thus, those who might most benefit are most resistive to increased activity. This view is reinforced by the fact that among family members (The General Mills American Family Report, 1978-1979), 15% smoke and do not intend to quit, 20% have tried but failed to quit, but only 16% report quitting successfully. Similarly, although 50% view overweight as a serious health threat, only 25% are consciously attempting to reduce caloric intake.

Although family members over 65 years of age and those between 18 and 34 are most likely to be regular exercisers (The General Mills American Family Report, 1978-1979), age is a direct influence on leisure activity levels across the general population (Harris and Associates, 1978). The energy requirements of leisure can be expected to drop by 15% in a linear fashion from age 20 to age 65 (Montoye, 1975). Age does not, however, predict adherence to clinical exercise programs (Dishman, 1982; Morgan, 1977; Oldridge, 1982).

Summary and Future Priorities

It appears clear that the health-promoting potential of physical activity and exercise cannot be determined until the behavioral determinants of participation are better understood and managed, yet, these remain poorly defined when viewed either from a narrow view of clinical exercise or from the encompassing perspective of public health. It has also become clear that attempts to explain exercise participation in supervised preventive medicine programs likely cannot advance in a systematic way until exercise behavior in other settings and population segments is more precisely described and understood. The indeterminance of existing knowledge points to the need for an upgrading of research methods in the study of exercise adherence.

Surveys with the most generalizable significance for public health rely on recall and subjective estimates of uncertain precision both for activity patterns and for a restricted set of behavioral influences; they may often appear to yield behaviorally incongruous results and not to permit relative weighting of influence. Better-controlled clinical and community studies have employed comparatively precise measures of behavior and independent variables in more interactive analyses, but their generalizability across populations, environments, and activity modes is limited. Although segregated in purpose, methods, and scope, current approaches do converge in implicating several common factors that are testable. However, experimental studies have largely manipulated behavior control principles and techniques, independent of personal and environmental

Table 9   A Process Approach

Knowledge/skills

Intention

The idea/the mood

Commitment

Reinforcement

---

characteristics shown to be related to activity patterns. Future study should resolve these disparities.

Regular participation must be viewed as a dynamic process in which adoption and maintenance are key outcomes, influenced by a person's health and behavioral traits related to willingness and ability to be active. Table 9 suggests key process concepts for experimental study. When these are viewed within the model presented earlier in Table 2, a more theoretical view of exercise behavior begins to emerge, which may help target important segments of the population and key behavioral factors in future intervention strategies for increasing participation and retarding the present dropout rates.

Although for many people regular participation must be a self-regulated behavior, initial adoption can be influenced by anticipation of a favorable benefit/cost evaluation. Prompting from agencies and health care professions highlighting benefits can influence adoption among the inactive, but the influence of prior intention to be active or prior activity history in mediating this effect remains unstudied. To maintain involvement effectively, socially-based support should be in the form of personalized encouragement and reinforcement delivered on an intermittent, but continuing, basis by health care providers, family, and peers. A predominant focus on health education is ineffective in promoting exercise among most adults, although it may facilitate moderate activity among the middle-aged and elderly. The psychological and epidemiologic impact of various activity modes and intensities, however, remains undetermined for these groups. The provision of facilities and supervision are perceived as important in older, but not younger, age groups. The key for many to maintain participation, however, seems to lie in concrete feelings of well-being, not in abstract fears about poor health or promises of longevity. In researchers' focus on why people drop out, they have largely neglected this important aspect of intrinsic reinforcement. To conclude merely that the active enjoy being active does little to explain why, and fails to show how to create this feeling in the inactive.

Study Recommendations

The following suggestions for future study and program evaluation are offered:

(a) Collectively, perceived barriers appear less influential in impeding participation than does lack of motivation. The actual importance of time, schedule and location convenience or flexibility, preferred activity modes and intensities, peer or family support and involvement, activity leadership styles, and the advice of medical and health care providers should be experimentally examined.

(b) The time course of effects from behavior modification strategies, and their underlying mechanisms, should be examined for client-centered behavior management techniques. Stimulus control, goal setting, and self-reinforcement techniques could be competitively contrasted with generalized social support.

(c) Naturally occurring intrinsic reinforcers related to an attitude of "feeling like being active" should be specified in biometric and psychometric terms. Personal monitoring and reinforcement skills underlying exercise commitment and self-motivation should be identified.

(d) The cognitive and behavioral-affective components of decision making, as they relate to intention to adopt an activity routine and ability to forestall or overcome relapse, should be investigated.

(e) It is not understood how and when preferences for types of physical activity or exertional levels are formed or what influence they exert on actual behavior patterns. The impact of genetic inheritance, peer and family influence, competitive sport, and physical education experience on these preferences should be examined.

(f) It is not known to what extent the failure to maintain involvement in various settings or activities influences, or is influenced by, attempts in other settings or activities. How previous successes and failures affect behavioral mediators also remains unexamined.

(g) Determining setting and activity interactions in exercise and other health behaviors appears critical in permitting an integrated effort in the study and support of exercise and physical fitness by clinical, community, commercial, and federal agencies. Standardization of study questions, variables, and measurement methods will be necessary, however, in examining the generalizability of behavior patterns across settings, activities, and population segments.

These recommendations and the public health perspective of the foregoing review are based on my belief that previous approaches to the study of exercise adherence, although logical and somewhat fruitful, have neared a point of diminishing returns in advancing either practically or

theoretically useful understandings of why people do or don't participate in exercise programs. The predominant early research focuses of
predicting adherence/dropout and modifying behavior through education or cognitive-behavioristic principles, while understandably pragmatic,
would probably be too short-sighted for future studies. We now need
to explain the process by which individuals decide (either rationally or
otherwise) to adopt and maintain regular exercise participation. I hope
my comments can help researchers frame more explanatory questions and
find more practically useful answers.

Meanwhile, I will presume to propose that the best long-term prescription for exercise adherence at the present time might be directed at those
of us who study health-related exercise. If just a portion of attention and
resources that have been directed at determining fitness were to be
directed at understanding exercise behavior, we might learn as much
about guidelines for promoting exercise adherence as we do about increasing $\dot{V}O_2$ max—in willing subjects!

References

Andrew, G.M., Oldridge, N.B., Parker, J.O., et al. (1981). Reasons for
dropout from exercise programs in post-coronary patients. *Medicine
and Science in Sports and Exercise, 13*, 164-168.

Blumenthal, J.A., Williams, R.S., Wallace, A.G., Williams, R.B., &
Needles, T.L. (1982). Physiological and psychological variables predict
compliance to prescribed exercise therapy in patients recovering from
myocardial infarction. *Psychosomatic Medicine, 6*, 519-527.

Brownell, L., & Stunkard, A.J. (1980). Physical activity in the development and control of obesity. In A.J. Stunkard (Ed.), *Obesity*. Philadelphia: Saunders.

Brownell, K., Stunkard, A.J., & Albaum, J. (1980). Evaluation and modification of exercise patterns in the natural environment. *American Journal of Psychiatry, 137*, 1540-1545.

Canada Fitness Survey. (1983). *Fitness and lifestyle in Canada*. Fitness and
Amateur Sport, Government of Canada, Ottawa, Ontario.

Clarke, H.H. (Ed.). (1973, May). National adult physical fitness survey.
President's Council on Physical Fitness and Sports Newsletter. Washington, DC.

Collingwood, T.R., Bernstein, I.H., & Hubbard, D. (1983). Caronical
correlation analysis of clinical and psychological data in 4,351 men
and women. *Journal of Cardiac Rehabilitation, 3*, 706-711.

Cox, M.H. (1984). Fitness and lifestyle programs for business and industry: Problems in recruitment and retention. *Journal of Cardiac Rehabilitation, 4*, 136-142.

Dishman, R.K. (1981a). Biologic influences on exercise adherence. *Research Quarterly for Exercise and Sport*, **52**, 143-159.

Dishman, R.K. (1981b). Prediction of adherence to habitual physical activity. In F.J. Nagle & H.J. Montoye (Eds.), *Exercise in health and disease*. Springfield, IL: Charles C Thomas.

Dishman, R.K. (1982). Compliance/adherence in health-related exercise. *Health Psychology*, **1**, 237-267.

Dishman, R.K. (1984). Motivation and exercise adherence. In J. Silva & R. Weinberg (Eds.), *Psychological foundations of sport*. Champaign, IL: Human Kinetics.

Dishman R.K. (1987). Exercise adherence and habitual physical activity. In W.P. Morgan & S.N. Goldston (Eds.), *Exercise and mental health* (pp. 57-83). Washington, DC: Hemisphere Publishing Corporation.

Dishman, R.K. (in press). Supervised and free-living physical activity: No differences in former athletes and nonathletes. *American Journal of Preventive Medicine*.

Dishman, R.K., & Ickes, W. (1981). Self-motivation and adherence to therapeutic exercise. *Journal of Behavioral Medicine*, **4**, 421-438.

Dishman, R.K., Sallis, J.F., & Orenstein, D. (1985). The determinants of physical activity and exercise. *Public Health Reports*, **100**, 158-171.

Epstein, L.H., Koeske, R., & Wing, R.R. (1984). Adherence to exercise in obese children. *Journal of Cardiac Rehabilitation*, **4**, 185-195.

Fielding, J.E. (1982). Effectiveness of employee health improvement programs. *Journal of Occupational Medicine*, **24**, 907-916.

Fitness Ontario: Blue collar workers and physical activity. (1981a). Toronto: Government of Ontario, Ministry of Culture and Recreation. Sports and Fitness Branch.

Fitness Ontario: Low active adults, who they are, how to reach them. (1981b). Government of Ontario, Ministry of Culture and Recreation. Sports and Fitness Branch.

Fitness Ontario: The relationship between physical activity and other health-related lifestyle beahviors. (1982). Toronto: Government of Ontario, Ministry of Culture and Recreation, Sports and Fitness Branch.

Franklin, B.A. (1978). Motivating and educating adults to exercise: Practical suggestions to increase interest and enthusiasm. *Journal of Physical Education and Recreation*, **49**, 13-17.

The General Mills American Family Report, 1978-1979: Family health in an era of stress. Yankelovich, Skelly and White, Inc.

Gettman, L.R., Pollock, M.L., & Ward, A. (1983). Adherence to unsupervised exercise. *The Physician and Sportsmedicine*, **11**(10), 56-66.

Gould, D., & Horn, D. (1984). Participation motivation in young athletes. In J. Silva & R. Weinberg (Eds.), *Psychological foundations in sport and exercise*. Champaign, IL: Human Kinetics.

Greendorfer, S.L. (1983). Family influences on sport. In M. Boutslier and SanGiovani (Eds.), *The sporting woman* (pp. 135-155). Champaign, IL: Human Kinetics.

Harris, D.V. (1970). Physical activity history and attitudes of middle-aged men. *Medicine and Science in Sports, 2*, 203-208.

King, A.L., & Frederiksen, L.W. (1984). Low-cost strategies for increasing exercise behavior: Relapse preparation training and social support. *Behavior Modification, 8*, 3-21.

LaPorte, R.E., Adams, L.L., Savage, D.D. et al. (1984). The spectrum of physical activity, cardiovascular disease and health: An epidemiologic perspective. *American Journal of Epidemiology, 120*, 507-517.

Lindsay-Reid, E., & Osborn, R.W. (1980). Readiness for exercise adoption. *Social Science and Medicine, 14*, 139-146.

Lobstein, D.D., Mosbacher, B.J., & Ismail, A.H. (1983). Depression as a powerful discriminator between physically active and sedentary middle-aged men. *Journal of Psychosomatic Research, 27*, 69-76.

Loy, J.W., McPherson, B., & Kenyon, G. (1978). *Sport and social systems*. Philadelphia: Saunders.

Marlatt, G.A., & Gordon, J.R. (1980). Determinants of relapse: Implications for the maintenance of behavior change. In P. Davidson & S. Davidson (Eds.), *Behavioral medicine: Changing health lifestyles*. New York: Brunner-Mazel.

Martin, J.E., & Dubbert, P.M. (1982). Exercise applications and promotion in behavioral medicine: Current status and future directions. *Journal of Consulting Clinical Psychology, 50*, 1004-1017.

Martin, J.E., Dubbert, P.M., Katell, A.D., Thompson, J.K., Raczynski, J.R., Lake, M., Smith, P.O., Webster, J.S., Sikova, T., & Cohen, R.E. (1984). The behavioral control of exercise in sedentary adults: Studies 1 through 6. *Journal of Consulting Clinical Psychology, 52*, 795-811.

McIntosh, P. (1980). *"Sport for All" programs throughout the world*. Report prepared for UNESCO (Contract No. 207604). New York: UNESCO.

Meyer, A., Nash, J., McAlister, A., Maccoby, N., & Farquhar, J.W. (1980). Skills training in a cardiovascular health education campaign. *Journal of Consulting Clinical Psychology, 48*, 129-142.

The Miller Lite report on American attitudes toward sports. (1983). New York: Research & Forecasts, Inc.

Montoye, H.J. (1975). *Physical activity and health: An epidemiological study of an entire community*. Englewood Cliffs, NJ: Prentice-Hall.

Montoye, H.J., Van Huss, W.P., Olson, H., Pierson, W.R., & Hudec, A. (1957). *Longevity and morbidity of college athletes*. Indianapolis: Phi Epsilon Kappa.

Morgan, W.P. (1977). Involvement in vigorous physical activity with special reference to adherence. In G.I. Gedvilas & M.E. Kneer (Eds.),

National College Physical Education Association Proceedings. Chicago: University of Illinois Press.

Morgan, W.P. (1979). Negative addiction in runners. *The Physician and Sportsmedicine,* **7**, 57-70.

Neilsen Poll. (1983). Statistical Report.

Oldridge, N.B. (1977). What to look for in an exercise class leader. *The Physician and Sportsmedicine,* **5**, 85-88.

Oldridge, N.B. (1982). Compliance and exercise in primary and secondary prevention of coronary heart disease: A review. *Preventive Medicine,* **11**, 56-70.

Oldridge, N.B., Donner, A., Buck, C.W. et al. (1983). Predictive indices for dropout: The Ontario Exercise Heart Collaborative Study experience. *American Journal of Cardiology,* **51**, 70-74.

Oldridge, N.B., & Jones, N.L. (1983). Improving patient compliance in cardiac rehabilitation effects of written agreement and self-monitoring. *Journal of Cardiac Rehabilitation,* **3**, 257-262.

Pandolf, K. (1983). Perceived exertion. In R. Terjung (Ed.), *Exercise and sport sciences reviews* (Vol. II). Philadelphia: Franklin Institute Press.

The Perrier Study: Fitness in America. Louis Harris and Associates, 1979.

Pollock, M.L., Gettman, L.R., Milesis, C.A., Beh, M., Durstine, L., & Johnson, M. (1977). Effects of frequency and duration of training on attrition and incidence of injury. *Medicine and Science in Sports,* **9**, 31-36.

Powell, K.E., & Dysinger, W. (in press). Childhood participation in organized school sports as precursors of adult physical activity. *American Journal of Preventive Medicine.*

Rejeski, W.J., Morley, D., & Miller, H.S. (1984). The Jenkins Activity Survey: Exploring its relationship with compliance to exercise prescription and MET gain within a cardiac rehabilitation setting. *Journal of Cardiac Rehabilitation,* **4**, 90-94.

Sacks, M.H., & Sachs, M.L. (Eds.). (1981). *Psychology of running.* Champaign, IL: Human Kinetics.

Sallis, J.F., Haskell, W.L., Fortmann, S.P., Vranizan, K.M., Taylor, C.B., & Soloman, D.S. (1986). Predictors of adoption and maintenance of physical activity in a community sample. *Preventive Medicine,* **15**, 331-341.

Shephard, R.J. (1978). *Physical activity and aging.* London: Croom Helm.

Shephard, R.J., Corey, P., & Kavanaugh, T. (1981). Exercise compliance and the prevention of recurrence of myocardial infarction. *Medicine and Science in Sports and Exercise,* **13**, 1-5.

Shephard, R.J., & Cox, M. (1980). Some characteristics of participants in an industrial fitness programme. *Canadian Journal of Applied Sport Science,* **5**(2), 69-76.

Sonstroem, R.J. (1982). Attitudes and beliefs in the prediction of exercise participation. In R.L. Cantu & W.J. Gillespie (Eds.) *Sports medicine, sports science: Bridging the gap.* Lexington, MA: The Collamore Press.

U.S. Department of Health and Human Services Prevention. 1982. Public Health Service, Office of Disease Prevention and Health Promotion. DHHS (PHS) Publication No. 82-50157. Washington, DC: U.S. Government Printing Office.

U.S. National Center for Health Statistics. (1980). *Health, United States 1977-1978*. Washington, DC: Department of Health and Human Services, US Government Printing Office.

Wankel, L.M. (1984). Decision-making and social-support strategies for increasing exercise involvement. *Journal of Cardiac Rehabilitation, 4*, 124-135.

Ward, A., & Morgan, W.P. (1984). Adherence patterns of healthy men and women enrolled in an adult exercise program. *Journal of Cardiac Rehabilitation, 4*, 143-152.

The approach to this chapter was aided greatly by my work on a similar review for the Centers for Disease Control, Atlanta, GA. I would like to acknowledge the contributions of Kenneth E. Powell, MD, Chief of the Behavioral Epidemiology and Evaluation Branch, in helping guide my perspective of exercise adherence toward the public health domain. This perspective should help us define program-related behavior in a clear and more meaningful way. Discussions with James F. Sallis, PhD, and Diane Orenstein, PhD, have also been useful.

Part II

The Model: Testing, Prescription, and Exercise in Chronic Disease

Chapter 6

The Basics of Exercise Prescription

Linda K. Hall

Often when conducting a workshop on exercise testing and exercise prescription, I am asked for a formula for writing the ideal exercise prescription for anyone. However, everyone is different, not only in shape and size, but also in response to stress, strain, and physical exercise. Therefore, it is essential to learn how to gather all of the available data relative to an individual's response to exercise stress, and then to apply them to accepted guidelines for prescribing exercise.

Who is Being Tested for the Prescription?

The "who" of the exercise prescription is more important than many people realize. Background and lifestyle information should be gathered before designing the exercise prescription and program. The questions in Appendix A need to be asked before proceeding to the next stage of gathering information and prescribing.

The next thing to ascertain is the degree of wellness (or sickness) of the person for whom you are prescribing. For the intent of this chapter an adult will be considered as any person at least 18 years old. Generally anyone under the age of 45 and apparently healthy should check with a physician to see whether there is any reason not to exercise, then fill out a Risk Factor Analysis Questionnaire and the PAR-Q Validation Report that appears in Appendix B (1985). A healthy adult under 45 who meets the criteria of the third edition of the American College of Sports Medicine (ACSM) Guidelines (1986) may begin an exercise program without exercise testing. Exercise prescription for such a person will be explained later.

Anyone above the age of 35 with higher risk by the ACSM criteria should have a physician-supervised maximal exercise test (GXT) prior to beginning a program of exercise. A high-risk individual is defined as one who has one or more of the following major risk factors: blood pressure higher than 140/90, a lipid profile ratio higher than 5, history of cigarette smoking, diabetes mellitus, and a member of their family (blood relation) who has manifested heart disease and/or atherosclerotic complications prior to the age of 50. However, an exercise test is not necessary for anyone below the age of 35. Yet, caution is emphasized in the beginning of any exercise program, as will be discussed later in this chapter.

A person with a diagnosed acute or chronic disease should be referred by a physician, should have available a medical history with facts pertinent to the effects of physiology and pathology on exercise parameters, and should have had a recent (within the last 3 months) GXT that was supervised by a physician. There should be a list of the amount and types of medications being taken by the patient, as well as any others taken when the GXT was performed. Also, there should not have been any changes in physical, anatomical, or pathological conditions which might have altered the outcome of the test had they been present when it was performed. There should be interpretations of the electrocardiogram (ECG) and other physiological parameters written by the physician. This is critical, especially if the patient has had a medication change since the test that would alter the heart rate (HR), blood pressure (BP), or other measurable parameters in response to exercise.

For example, suppose that a 50-year-old person is tested while on a daily prescription of 40 milligrams (mg) of Inderal. Though one might expect to see a slow and blunted response of heart rate to exercise, the person could achieve a maximum heart rate of 150 during testing. Suppose also that as a result of the test, the physician increases the prescription of Inderal to 100 mg per day and does not retest. You, the exercise specialist, now have no indication of what will happen to heart rate and blood pressure as a result of increased beta-blocking effects. You might give a heart rate prescription for exercise that the person simply cannot achieve, forcing an effort which could bring about disasterous results.

What You Can Glean From the Exercise Test

Two important factors, among many, gleaned from exercise tests are maximal exercise capacity and maximal functional capacity. We will examine both of these factors and their impact on the exercise prescription in more detail.

Maximal Exercise Capacity and
Maximal Functional Capacity

Determination of maximal exercise capacity usually requires the combination of many possible factors. The most specific determination would result when the test is performed not only with an ECG and a heart rate and blood pressure monitor, but also with a metabolic assessment of oxygen uptake, maximal exercise capacity being indicated when the usually accepted parameters for maximum work are achieved. These parameters include heart rate plateauing, oxygen consumption plateauing or not increasing as work increases, respiratory quotient (RQ) of greater than 1.0, and a volitional termination of the test by the testee.

However, in the case of the usual procedure used with graded exercise testing, a protocol is chosen with progressing workloads that have been tested, with estimated oxygen utilization predicted. When this is the case, maximal exercise tolerance is that point at which one or all of the following occur: (a) the patient volitionally terminates the test because he feels that he cannot go any further, (b) a symptom occurs which the physician feels is ominous or limiting, or (c) the patient develops a symptom which is limiting to his or her sense of ability to exercise and does not wish to continue. It is important to note the procedure among physicians in the laboratory doing the exercise testing. Several examples of things important to know when determining what is maximal exercise and what is functional maximal exercise capacity are listed below:

- Some physicians utilize the simple formula "220 minus age" as the predictor of maximal heart rate; when the person being tested achieves that rate, the test is terminated, whether it is true max or not. The formula is at best only an estimation and has as one standard deviation ± 10 beats per minute (bpm).
- Some physicians will consider 1 millimeter (mm) of S-T depression as the time when a test should be concluded, but others will push patients beyond that level until true maximal capacity occurs.
- Physicians may consider a rating of perceived exertion (RPE) of 17 as maximal capacity. Others, as was the case in a hospital in which I worked, would push the patient to a 20, and only after having described a 20 as working at such an intense effort that even if your barn was burning down with 80 of your prized heifers in it, you would let it burn.

Maximal functional capacity is that point at which a symptom is either expressed by the patient (shortness of breath, leg pain, chest pain, dizziness, etc.) or manifested on the ECG (S-T depression, PVCs, SVT, some other ECG abnormalities), there is a plateauing of heart rate, or blood pressure rises or falls abnormally. Maximal functional capacity is an indication of that point at which healthy response to exercise terminates and pathology manifests itself. The physician and the patient may agree to go on, or the physician may pursue the test further if the patient is unaware of his abnormal response.

The final point at which the test is terminated is the maximal exercise capacity. Let me here emphasize the difference between functional max and maximal exercise capacity. Functional max is that point in the test at which pathology shows either objective ECG, BP, or HR changes or subjective pain, claudication, shortness of breath (SOB), etc.; it is not necessarily the point at which the test is ended. Maximal exercise capacity *is* that point at which the test ends (unless it is determined to be a 75% or 85% of max test).

Prescription Rule #1: Exercise is prescribed using the reference point of maximal functional capacity, with the identifying parameters of heart rate, MET level, RPP, and/or RPE as markers of that point. This might be the same as maximal exercise capacity if the test is terminated with no symptoms other than fatigue, or if the test is terminated at the first sign of symptoms.

Heart Rate and Blood Pressure Response

In a healthy response to exercise, the heart rate peaks and flattens, the blood pressure and O_2 uptake rise linearly, peak, flatten, and might even drop a little; and the person taking the test determines that he/she can not go on. Figure 1 demonstrates a composite of normal heart rate and blood pressure response in relation to duration and metabolic workload. Occasionally there will be an immediate rise in HR and BP, then a slight dip, then a linear rise again until maximal values are attained. This immediate rise, which is often a bit oversized, is usually the result of apprehension over the test, treadmill noise, 10 electrodes, a new machine, personnel, which can all give rise to a nervous response in the best of people.

Heart rate is closely related to cardiac reserve (increased potential for more work by the heart), fitness level, general health, sinus node function, and various other elements, such as temperature and humidity. However, the most important factor in heart rate response is age; as one grows older, the ability of the heart to increase its rate decreases (note the use of the predictor of 220 minus age as heart rate maximum). When the heart rate response is less than normal, level of endurance training, sinus node dysfunction, ventricular dysfunction (inotropic incompetence leading to chronotropic incompetence), and medications should be taken into account. With sinus node dysfunction, other symptoms such as diz-

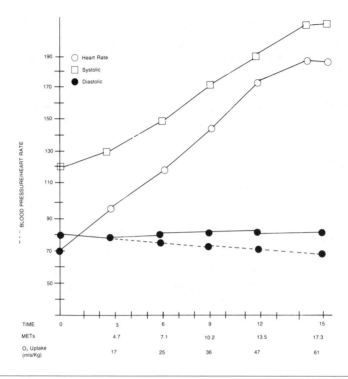

Figure 1 This figure demonstrates a composite of normal heart rate and blood pressure responses in relation to duration and/or metabolic work load.

ziness, SOB, and possibly dysrhythmias usually manifest themselves (Abbott, 1977). Chronotropic incompetence is a blunted heart rate response to exercise, indicating ventricular contractibility dysfunction and carrying a portent of a coronary event or sudden death (Ellested & Wan, 1975; Hinkle, Carver, & Plankun, 1972; Jose & Taylor, 1969).

Blood pressure is an important parameter in exercise response. Diastolic pressure should stay the same or, in response to decreasing peripheral resistance, fall more than 10 mmHg. Diastolic blood pressure rising is often a response of people with coronary artery disease (Sheps et al., 1979). Do not be alarmed if diastolic is heard all the way to zero, even though muffled. It is normal and not a sign of dysfunction. Systolic blood pressure should rise linearly, fall off at maximal levels, drop off immediately after maximal exercise is obtained and cool-down is started, rise again, and then steadily decline to normal. Blood pressure falling before maximal effort is achieved usually indicates critical coronary artery disease. Make sure that there are accompanying symptoms and that a proper check is made before assuming the fall is correct (Morris & McHenry, 1977).

Prescription Rule #2: That point at which there is a major change in heart rate progression (flattening, drop, failure to rise with increasing workloads, etc.), systolic blood pressure (rapid rise to hypertensive levels, drop of 10 mmHg or more before maximal exercise is achieved), or diastolic blood pressure (increase in pressure greater than 10 mmHg) shall be considered maximal functional exercise capacity; prescription of exercise will be made at a level below that.

Electrocardiographic Responses

This is the part of the exercise test which is to be read and interpreted by a cardiologist or qualified physician. There are a number of things which are to be considered when interpreting arrhythmias and S-T segment elevation or depression. Suffice it to say that if questions arise regarding the significance of the depression or arrhythmias, do not proceed on the assumption that they are benign, unless so signified in writing by a physician. Figure 2 illustrates the classic forms of exercise-induced S-T segment depression (Rijneke, 1980). The point of appearance of these is indicative of maximal functional capacity.

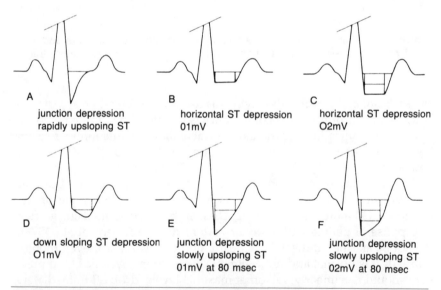

A   junction depression
    rapidly upsloping ST

B   horizontal ST depression
    01mV

C   horizontal ST depression
    02mV

D   down sloping ST depression
    01mV

E   junction depression
    slowly upsloping ST
    01mV at 80 msec

F   junction depression
    slowly upsloping ST
    02mV at 80 msec

Figure 2 Different types of exercise-induced S-T segment depression, including three forms of J-junction depression (*A, E* and *F*). *Note.* From "Clinical Significance of Upsloping S-T Segments in Exercise Electrocardiography" by R.D. Rijneke et al., 1980, *Circulation,* **61**, p. 671. Copyright 1980 by the American Heart Association, Inc. Reprinted by permission of the American Heart Association, Inc.

Prescription Rule #3. The appearance of interpreted S-T segment depression (as illustrated in Figure 2) shall be the determinant of functional maximal capacity; prescription of exercise will be made at a level below that.

Arrythmias are another case altogether and definitely require consultation with the physician in charge of the patient. There are forms of benign and malignant arrhythmias other than those that are obvious. Everyone sometime in the day has an isolated PVC or two; however, beyond that, form and number must be interpreted by the physician. There can be no rule about the point in the test at which arrhythmias arrive, for it has been demonstrated numerous times that reproducibility is a variable item ranging from 14% (Fabian, Stolz, Janota, & Rohac, 1975) to 100% (Rozanski, Dimich, Steinfeld, & Kupersmith, 1979) at any time, depending upon methods used and types of subjects studied.

Generally, if arrhythmia has been picked up on ECG, the physician is aware of it and has made a determination whether to medicate for it. With the recent advent of electrophysiological studies, arrhythmias are well in hand, and the physician has made appropriate notation, when the patient arrives for exercise prescription. However, if a new pattern develops at any time during exercise, specifically while you are monitoring or the patient comments, exercise should cease; the physician should be notified immediately. In patients stress-tested upon discharge from the hospital, arrhythmias, specifically ventricular ectopy, will show up in 20-60% of the patients. Approximately 25% of these will normalize within the next 6 weeks. However, 33% of those tested with no abnormality at discharge will manifest one within the next 6 weeks (Fagin, Wayne, & McConachy, 1984).

Prescription Rule #4: Appearance of a new form of arrhythmia during exercise in any participant means exercise should be brought to a progressive halt; the patient should be seated and monitored, and a strip should be run, during the arrhythmia. Other evident symptoms should be noted, blood pressure taken, and all strips and parameters reported to the physician at this time. The patient should not be released from your care until directed to be so by the physician.

Other Parameters, Observed and Measured

Length of time on a treadmill or bicycle is an excellent measure to aid in prescribing exercise. The longer the patient is on the machine, the better the prognosis for tolerance and baseline conditioning. If the length of time is very short, check whether the protocol chosen was appropriate for the age, sex, and condition of the patient. Sometimes physicians use the standard Bruce protocol, and patients, especially deconditioned women, will be at more than half of their exercise tolerance in the first stage. At such a high intensity, an inappropriate warm-up occurs and S-T depression appears, which might bring about a false positive conclusion to the test. In some cases it would be better to have done a GXT that assesses length of time on the treadmill with slow progressing workloads, rather than a quickie with no helpful information from which to make an excellent prescription (Hall, 1987). It is precisely this possible outcome that makes it essential to determine the type of test—functional, diagnostic, or discharge—being done in order to select a protocol which elicits the kind of response needed.

> **Prescription Rule #5**: Make note of the length of time the patient was able to stay on the modality during the test; utilize this set point for length of time for endurance activity during exercise training.

Appearance of cyanosis around the mouth and nails is an ominous indication of pump dysfunction. Inappropriate skin response upon blanching also alerts you to heart problems. These should be noted on the test; the point of arrival of these symptoms is a significant indication of functional maximal ability. Shortness of breath is an indicator of respiratory distress. The point at which it is noted by the patient is indicative of functional maximal ability. People in good health experience this point at about the same time that all other parameters are maximizing. People with a pathology related to the cardiorespiratory system manifest it earlier than maximal ability and explain that it makes exercise stressful. It is a point below which exercise should be prescribed.

Subjective Data From the Patient

Quizzing patients during testing about how they feel gives information relative to dizziness, claudication, and the appearance of angina. Each one of these in itself is an indication of functional maximal capacity, the time of onset should be duly noted. The heart rate and blood pressure as well as an ECG strip should also be recorded at the onset of chest pain to see whether the pain is manifested together with ischemia.

The heart rate and blood pressure utilized together in the form of a rate pressure product (RPP) indicates the level of myocardial oxygen supply (RPP is often referred to as "double product" in the literature). It has been noted that angina and ischemia are not reproducible at a specific speed, grade, heart rate, or blood pressure. However, they are reproducible at the same rate pressure product. Calculation of rate pressure product is as follows:

$$\frac{\text{Heart rate} \times \text{Systolic Blood Pressure}}{100}$$

The number arrived at has no units and is merely an indication, in this case, of the point at which ischemia and angina manifest themselves. As training in exercise endurance progresses, it takes longer and more intense work for that RPP to be achieved or angina or ischemia to appear (Ellestad, 1980).

Prescription Rule #6: Make note of the rate pressure product at which angina or ischemia appears. This is also a functional maximal capacity point, and exercise should be prescribed below it.

Medications

It is important for the exercise prescriber and administrator to understand the effects of medications on heart rate, blood pressure, ischemia, and length of exercise duration. Certain medications, such as the beta-blockers, blunt heart rate and blood pressure response. Sometimes this blunting can be so extreme that the patient does not manifest any more than a one- or two-beat change from rest through warm-up, exercise, and cooldown. This should be understood and duly noted. Some tests are read as positive from an S-T segment depression perspective, when in fact the S-T segment problem was present at rest and was a result of digitalis preparation. There are numerous published manuals with information relative to the medication effects of each drug on exercise tolerance, BP, HR, and ECG. One of these manuals should be a part of the GXT lab and exercise area. Another one that should be available at all times and utilized for all medications before making and implementing a prescription for exercise is the most current issue of the *Physicians Desk Reference* (PDR).

Concluding Remarks to Section I

This section has brought to light many of the parameters fitness specialists overlooked when prescribing exercise. It is essential that exercise prescribed is tolerable both physiologically and anatomically to the patient. It is always better to underprescribe when in doubt, but careful inspection of the GXT and all of the above-mentioned parameters will give a much better platform from which to build an exacting prescription.

Prescription Rule #7: Do not prescribe exercise at a level at which the participant experiences pain, arrhythmias, or any sensation likely to induce fear or anxiety. People will only participate in things that are pleasantly stimulating—not exhausting—and from which they can recover easily.

The Components of the Exercise Program and Prescription

Now that all of the participant's background information—pathology, capacity, physiological and anatomical parameters—has been collected and examined, actual exercise prescription can begin. First though, there are a few terms that should be defined in order for the prescription to be done well.

$\dot{V}O_2$ **Max: Maximal Aerobic Power** is the maximal amount of oxygen that the body can take in, take up, transport, and give to working tissue for use in metabolism to produce energy for work. It may be expressed several ways: absolutely in liters of oxygen utilized per minute of work. This does not make it a valuable tool for individualizing the value. If two people each utilize 2 liters of oxygen per minute, are you able to distinguish which one is more fit? When the value is expressed in relative terms, per unit of body weight for example, one is then able to make comparisons to norms and other performances. Thus a relative expression of maximal oxygen uptake would be in milliliters per kilogram body weight or mls/Kg-body weight per minute. Another way of expressing maximal oxygen uptake is in mls/Kg-lean body weight with fat weight subtracted out.

MET is an average value for resting oxygen consumption while sitting idly in a chair. Having measured a large number of people and calculated the average value to be 3.5 mls O_2/Kg-body weight-minute, work, exercise, and activities are valued at specific MET levels which means that they can be described in multiples of resting values. For example: climbing a flight of stairs is measured as taking 7-9.5 mls O_2/Kg to produce the energy needed or from 2-3 METs or valued as 2-3 times harder than sitting idly in a chair; see Table 1 for the four generally accepted ranges used to describe fitness and performance.

Functional Aerobic Impairment (FAI) is defined as the amount of disability a person has in percentage of what is the expected normal. It is calculated by taking a predicted value of performance for age and conditioning, subtracting the achieved value and dividing by the expected predicted value, multiplying by 100 to achieve a percentage. If the final value is subtracted from 100, the resulting number is the percentage of

Table 1   Variable MET Levels

Descriptor	MET Level
Limited	$\leqslant 6$
Asymptomatic/deconditioned	7-10
Healthy active	11-15
Endurance athlete	$\geqslant 16$

Table 2   Prediction Equations for $\dot{V}O_2$ Max for Healthy Men and Women

Group	Predicted $\dot{V}O_2$ Max
Active men	69.7 − .612 (age in years)
Sedentary men	57.8 − .445 (age in years)
Active women	42.9 − .312 (age in years)
Sedentary women	42.3 − .356 (age in years)

Note.

$$FAI = \frac{\text{Predicted } \dot{V}O_2 \text{ Max} - \text{Achieved } \dot{V}O_2 \text{ Max}}{\text{Predicted } \dot{V}O_2 \text{ Max}} \times 100$$

From "Principles of Exercise Testing" by R.A. Bruce, 1973, in J.P. Naughton and H.K. Hellerstein (Eds.), *Exercise Testing and Exercise Training in Coronary Heart Disease*, New York: Academic Press. Copyright 1973 by Academic Press. Reprinted by permission.

normal that the person is capable of achieving in terms of energy production and work effort. See Table 2 for prediction equations used to determine FAI for active and sedentary men and women.

Rate Pressure Product (RPP) is an expression and estimation of oxygen demand by the myocardium. It is the heart rate multiplied by systolic blood pressure, divided by 100. There are no units of expression and it is a linearly increasing value as work increases and myocardial oxygen demand increases. At maximal work numbers should fall into the following categories. If they don't it is an indication that the myocardium is not receiving the oxygen needed to function optimally.

Men   Values = to or above 325
Women   Values = to or above 285

Aerobic/Anaerobic are two terms which essentially mean with and without oxygen, respectively. They are descriptive terms for the way in which food substrates are broken down to produce the energy component (ATP) for the body's work. Anaerobic work is that work which is done in a high power, speed type effort which lasts up to a minute to a minute and a half, is fairly exhaustive from an effort point of view and produces a by-product, lactic acid. The lactic acid is removed during recovery from the exercise through four possible mechanisms: urine and sweat, conversion to glucose/glycogen, conversion to protein, and oxidation. Anaerobic work is not considered a cardiorespiratory fitness producer and has not been indicated as a resource for improving fitness, longevity, respiratory and cardiac efficiency, oxygen transport and/or exchange.

Aerobic work is an endurance activity which uses oxygen in the production of ATP. It is a pay-as-you-go system; leaves no waste products; and can function as long as there are food substrates to fuel it, the nervous system can tolerate the stress, and boredom does not overcome the exerciser. This energy system produces cardio-respiratory efficiency, improved oxygen uptake, improved fitness, and all of the benefits associated with wellness, health, and longevity.

Anaerobic Threshold (AT) is a term used to indicate that point during work when metabolism starts a transition into energy production that is anaerobic in nature. Current training theory for producing maximum aerobic endurance is to work at an effort just under that threshold. It usually occurs at about 75% of HR max, between 65-70% of $\dot{V}O_2$ max, and an RPE of about 14 or 15.

Rating of Perceived Exertion (RPE) is a method of subjectively evaluating the degree of difficulty of the task that is being performed. As established by Borg (1970) it is a scale ranging from 6 (very, very light) to 20 (very, very hard) which rates the intensity of the work effort and correlates well with training intensities.

Total Fitness Program (TFP) is one which includes all of the aspects of exercise to meet the total requirements for optimum physical, anatomical and physiological health: Warm up, cool down, aerobic exercise, strength and flexibility.

These terms will be interspersed with the prescriptive information and will make it easier to understand the factors being described and how they interact with the prescriptive process.

The next section will try to answer the most basic questions asked in workshops on exercise prescription. They are probably the most important questions you will consider when working with your patients.

What Type of Exercise Program Is Appropriate?

This aspect of exercise prescription depends upon who is receiving the prescription. If this participant has no health limitations, it is necessary only to find activities that will serve as an enjoyable, lifetime TFP. If you are working with a recently discharged post-mycardial infarction or CABG, angina, deconditioned, CAD, or COPD patient, a specially designed program with specified modalities is best for the first 8-15 weeks. Table 3 lists all types of exercises at varying MET levels that may be used as part of the exercise program. Fitting together exercises that the person likes to do and that meet the strength, endurance, and flexibility requirements is perhaps the hardest part. That it is important for participants to enjoy the activities is obvious: If people like to do something, they will be eager to do it; if they don't like to do something, they will postpone it indefinitely. Remember, you are trying to get the person involved for a lifetime.

Table 3   Activities and Their MET Values

1.0-2.9 METs	3.0-4.9 METs	5.0-6.9 METs
Walking 1.7 mph, flat	Walking 3.0 mph, flat	Walking 4.5 mph
Walking 2.0 mph, flat	Walking 4.0 mph, flat	Cycling 9.4 mph
Bicycle 50 rpms/.5Kg	Bicycle 50 rpms/1Kg	Cycling 50 rpms/2Kg
Golf, with power cart	Golf, walk and pull cart	Golf, carry clubs
Dancing, slow ballroom	Table tennis	Tennis, singles
Horseback, at a walk	Horseback, regular	Tennis, doubles
Canoeing, leisure	Swimming laps, easy	Swimming laps
	Backpacking, level	X-country skiing
	Rowing, stationary	Rowing, stationary
	Rowing, easy water	Rowing, water
	Weight lifting	Weight lifting
	Easy aerobics	Aerobic dance
	Badminton	Hunting

Prescription Rule #8: A program designed for any person wishing to pursue exercise should include all of the components required to achieve total fitness—warm up; work for flexibility, strength, and cardiorespiratory endurance; and cool-down. Table 3 is not an exclusive list. However, if you know the participant's functional maximal capacity and have decided upon the most suitable intensity, you should look in a reference work with activity listings (such as the one by McArdle, Katch, and Katch [1981]) to determine appropriate exercise.

Phase II Rehabilitation

A special comment about the modalities utilized in Phase II rehabilitation is needed here. Phase II is the period of time immediately after chronic disease patients are discharged from the hospital. The total time in the program varies from 8-15 weeks, depending upon such complicating factors as degree of deconditioning and adjustment to lifestyle change. It was formerly customary to spend most of the effort with these patients in a walking or bicycling program, improving cardiovascular condition. It is more apparent now that the majority of these people will return to work that entails more upper body than lower body demands. Another factor is that disease and reconditioning demand a whole-body effort, not only a lower body effort.

At the Christ Hospital, we work with six modalities, three for the upper body and three for the lower body, alternating the extremity regions. We try to encourage working a specific length of time (at least 15 minutes) continuously on one modality of choice (usually the treadmill or bicycle), then building to 10-minute components on the other apparatus. The choice of components are the personal preferences of the exercise specialists. Ours currently include the treadmill, bicycle ergometer, rowing machine, stairs, armcrank, and minigym wall pulley; we are about to add a 12-station weight machine to the program, as well as a Cybex UBE and Airdyne bicycles. The variety of experiences afforded once again enables the patient to find something pleasurable. For a more detailed explanation of the use of circuit training programming and upper arm work in a Phase II setting, refer to the work of Meyer (1984), Porter (1984), and Anderson (1987).

If your Phase II program is an at-home program in which the patient is responsible for daily exercise programming, you might wish to set up a situation in which your patients can lease rowing machines to get an upper body workout from rowing each day in addition to a lower body workout from walking. The saying that "variety is the spice of life" applies to exercise programming. This is why it is important to interview each of the people you will be working with as patients or participants to find out what they have done in the past and might want to do in the present and future.

We have become inventive with some of our at-home patients: We start with regular upper body calisthenics with small soup cans in each hand.

As their strength and conditioning increases, we increase the size of the cans and the number of repetitions. Some people who have their own exercise bicycles at home can ride the bicycles for lower leg work, sit behind the bicycles and pedal with their arms, walk, and use the cans— thus having a four-modality, at-home program relatively easily.

Exercise specialists sometimes ask: "Can chronic disease patients get back to doing what they have done before, or to what normal people do?" In about 50-60% of the cases of uncomplicated MI and CABG, the person can return to the level of activity that was a part of his/her lifestyle 10, 15, or 20 years earlier. Patients experience a loss of weight, a return of condition, and an increase of energy, becoming in many ways as fit as they were in their twenties. So, yes, they often can return to—and in some cases surpass—the lifestyles that their normal counterparts are enjoying.

Teaching the person how to prepare for involvement is the key to his or her resuming an active life. For example, at La Crosse in the Phase III program, we had a 42-year-old, post anterior wall MI, four-graft CABG patient. After a full 2 years of exercise conditioning, he wanted to go on a canoe trip into the Boundary Waters. We put a canoe into the swimming pool, paddled it, tipped it, swamped it, and had him fall out and climb back in. We spent time in the parking lot working on lifting, carrying, and portage skills. When he packed his gear, he took double sets of medications, his prescriptions, and a short medical record (the extra meds, the prescriptions, and the medical record were then kept in the guide's canoe). The man spent 6 days in the Boundary Waters, his only problem being poison ivy. He reported that his conditioning and strength were equal to at least half of the people there and better than another third—and some of those were younger men.

How Hard Should the Exercise Program Be?

This is an area which can become complicated, because of the myriad of methods, theories, and formulas. If the participant is a normal, healthy adult, the big question to ask is, "Why are you getting into exercise?" If 10K races and half-marathons are projected, serious exercise programming is required. If involvement is simply for the sake of good health, I recommend the KISS principle of difficulty—"Keep It Simple, Specialist!"

Talk/Sing Method of Exercise Prescription

Tell your patients: Never exercise so hard that you cannot talk in full sentences without gasping; if you gasp, you are exercising too hard. If you can sing with no difficulty, then you are not exercising hard enough. As you become conditioned, the work load increases with no apparent change; as talking becomes easier, increase effort.

Intensity Range

Professionals generally agree that the range of intensity can be as low as 40% and should not exceed 85% of the functional capacity. The low value of 40% is used with deconditioned or chronic disease persons who are in early recovery and, in some cases with elderly persons (American College of Sports Medicine, 1986; Franklin, Hellerstein, Gordon, & Timmis, 1986). No matter who is starting the exercise program, care should be taken in the initial stages of exercise.

> **Prescription Rule #9:** Along with warm-up exercises of about 5-10 minutes, preparing all of the joints and general musculoskeletal areas to be involved in the program, it is essential to start each major component of the program slowly and increase intensity in a gradual manner toward the target.

Reviewing all of the information gathered from the testing procedures and all of the parameters discussed earlier, you now have the tools to determine the intensity of the exercise you will prescribe. The following are all parameters that you may use in determining a scientifically derived exercise prescription.

Methods of Scientifically Prescribing Intensity

Heart Rate: What was the functional HR max attained? Has this person exercised in the past year? Is this person well-coordinated, or of average coordination? The less the experience with exercise, the lower the percentage of Karvonen HR reserve will be the prescription.

Karvonen HR reserve is the difference between resting and functional max HR (this is also called the "functional reserve") (Karvonen, Kentala, & Mustala, 1957). If resting HR is 70, and functional HR max is 170, then the reserve is 100 beats that can be utilized in increasing work. Multiply the percentage of work intensity desired times the heart rate reserve; add the resulting number to the resting heart rate. This is the HR prescription.

Example:		
Functional max HR	=	180 bpm
Resting heart rate	=	70 bpm
Reserve HR	=	110 bpm
Rx work intensity	=	.70
Rx beats	=	77 bpm
Resting HR	=	70 bpm
Exercise Rx HR	=	147 bpm

Using this method makes for a more accurate prescription of intensity of exercise and gives better training results than straight percentage of functional max HR. In this case, 70% of 180 equals a prescription HR of 126. Fitness might be attained with this HR only taking longer. An adjustment of this 126 bpm, by adding another 10-15% to the percentage when calculating percentage of functional max HR, can achieve the same fitness results much more quickly.

MET: Using MET level to determine exercise prescription is a marker tool for you as the prescriber, not a goal for the exerciser. There are very few people in the world who would know what to do if told to work at a 6 MET workload. However, in looking over the exercise test, you can determine the HR, RPE, and estimated functional $\dot{V}O_2$ max level. Franklin et al. (1986) have stated that optimal training occurs at intensities between 57% and 78% of $\dot{V}O_2$ max. Knowing the MET level achieved, determine exercise intensity by taking 60% of the MET level, plus METs/100. For example, suppose the functional max MET level achieved was 8; the prescription is $(0.60 + 8/100) \times 8$, equals 0.68×8, equals 5.4 METs. Look on the exercise test and see what the HR and RPE are at 5.4 METs; that will be the level of intensity in HR bpm or RPE. Table 4 gives you a sliding scale example of MET levels for conditioning.

Table 4   Physical Conditioning Intensities Using METs

Functional max MET Level	$0.60 + METs/100$ $(\dot{V}O_2/100)$	METs Rx Intensity
3	$0.60 + 0.03 = 0.63$	$(0.63 \times 3) = 1.90$
5	$0.60 + 0.05 = 0.65$	$(0.65 \times 5) = 3.25$
10	$0.60 + 0.10 = 0.70$	$(0.70 \times 10) = 7.00$
12	$0.60 + 0.12 = 0.72$	$(0.72 \times 12) = 8.64$

Rating of Perceived Exertion is an exceptionally useful tool for prescribing exercise for cardiac patients and other chronic disease patients who have heart rates blunted by medications. It is a good tool also because it encourages people to tune into what their bodies are telling them while working. Their intensity of breathing, sweating, muscle contraction, pace, and other feelings of work all give patients clues for the subjective evaluation of their exertion. People often are asked to rate things on a scale of 1-10, 1-100, and so on, so rating is not an unfamiliar task. People rate similar intensities with the same number on repeated trials. For chronic disease patients, a rating of 12-13 on the Borg scale (see Figure 3), which is equal to the description of "somewhat hard," gives a training intensity close to the upper limit of the exercise prescription. As the person

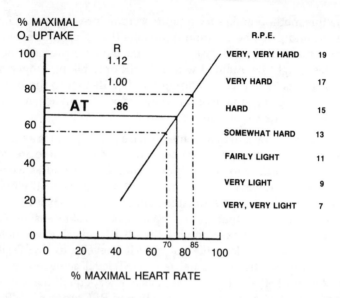

Figure 3 Relationships among percentage maximal oxygen uptake ($\dot{V}O_2$), percentage maximal heart rate (HR), respiratory exchange ratio (R), anaerobic threshold (AT), and Borg's rate of perceived exertion (RPE). The AT occurred at $\dot{V}O_2$ max (67.3% SE 1.78%) and HR max (75.5% SE 1.77) and R 0.86 SE .0087. The RPE of normal subjects and coronary patients did not differ significantly, 14.2 and 13.5 respectively; this corresponded to a rating between "somewhat hard" and "hard." *Note.* From "Exercise Testing and Prescription" by H.K. Hellerstein and B.A. Franklin, 1984, in N.H. Wenger and H.K. Hellerstein (Eds.), *Rehabilitation of the Coronary Patient* (p. 241). Copyright © 1984 by John Wiley and Sons, Inc. Reprinted by permission of John Wiley and Sons, Inc.

progresses toward a higher level of functional capacity, RPEs of 14 and 15 correspond to levels of 70-85% heart rate and 60-75% $\dot{V}O_2$ max.

In Figure 3 heart rate, METS, and RPE are graphically represented. The interrelationships of HR, RPE, and $\dot{V}O_2$ are demonstrated, and the percentages of functional max measurement of the parameters are also interwoven.

Prescription Rule #10: When prescribing "how hard," remember there is no *one* rule! There are many. My list follows.

Rule 10-1 For the chronic disease patient, never prescribe at an HR level that you have not seen on an ECG or at a level for which you have no cushion of beats above. This might mean that as you arrive during training at the functional max HR of the discharge GXT, it is necessary to give a ministress test to move the functional max HR higher.

Rule 10-2 For any patient or participant on whom you have a GXT with ECG record, never Rx a prescription HR above the highest recorded or without a cushion.

Rule 10-3 If you are prescribing for someone apparently healthy or under 35 with a major risk factor, but have no GXT data or ECG, a conservative Rx is best. No HR above 60% of estimated max HR (220 minus age) should be prescribed.

Rule 10-4 Make every effort to have your prescription HR, RPE, and METs align. For example, 60% of Karvonen HR reserve is comparable to 12-13 RPE, which is comparable to 52-54% of $\dot{V}O_2$ max.

Rule 10-5 Try to key the participant into reading how his body feels and how intense his breathing, sweat, and musculature coordination sensations are when at the levels of work you have prescribed.

Anaerobic Threshold

Figure 3 demonstrates the interrelationships of anaerobic threshold (AT) to $\dot{V}O_2$, HR, and RPE. I have not previously discussed AT in relation to exercise intensity because the type of participant who could find it important to train or exercise at that high level has not been the object of concern. However, once in a while you might come into contact with someone in a wellness program, industrial program, or, yes, even a rehabilitation program who wants a well-organized program in which to train for some serious timed 5K or 10K races. It is for this person that understanding the role of AT and intensity of training occurs.

In the definition of AT it is said that the best training effect for aerobic endurance takes place when work is done at a level just below the anaerobic threshold. This training level is one that borders the edge of pain, breathlessness, and a 15 RPE, one that increases heart rate and $\dot{V}O_2$ as endurance capacity improves. Alberto Salazar, running a 2-hour and 7-minute marathon, ran those 26-plus miles at close to a 13 mph pace, a heart rate of 180, a level of 85% of his maximal ability, and right at the AT level. For a person starting to work out using AT as his Rx, these kinds of numbers are impossible. For the new trainee using AT, the HR is likely to be 170, the RPE 15, and the percentage of $\dot{V}O_2$ max closer to 67%.

There is also the likelihood that unless the genes for superior aerobic physiological mechanisms are present, the new person will never get to Salazar's level. Having trained at the AT level, all of the parameters for increasing aerobic performance continue to be stretched to overload, producing increases in each system, each then responding to produce better performance.

Take caution when setting up a program that will lead to training work at AT. It is essential to start gradually. A low intensity should be prescribed until an aerobic base of cardiorespiratory endurance is present. Then slowly increase the percentage of Karvonen until AT training level is achieved. People will know that they are training around AT when, after slowly warming up and progressing into the endurance portion, they get up to a workload with an HR equal to 75% of HR reserve, an RPE of 14.5-15, and bordering on difficulty in talking evenly while working.

How Long and How Often Should Your Exerciser Work Out?

The best length and frequency of workouts depend upon the deconditioned level, pathology of disease, and past experience of the participant. Chronic disease patients need to exercise more frequently, but for shorter periods of time; for example, 15 minutes of walking once in the morning and once in the evening might be appropriate. Sometimes a COPD person might exercise 1 minute, rest 30 seconds, and repeat this pattern to achieve 5 minutes of exercise; the 5-minute workout is done four times per day.

For any healthy person, the base amount of time of continuous work at a submaximal heart rate needed to achieve a physiological fitness effect is 15 minutes. For the best effect, the intensity of the 15 minutes should eventually be quite taxing. However, people generally want neither to work very hard nor to devote a lot of time to an exercise program. Thus, the key is to get them started in an activity that is not over-demanding in time commitment, yet will be done long enough and often enough to produce the desired benefits. I ask people to give me 30 minutes of their time, 3 days a week; when they are able to commit to that and exercise regularly, they themselves probably want to increase the workout length and frequency.

If the people starting the program seem very eager and committed, start out slowly and increase gradually. Start with 5-10 minutes of warm-up, 20 minutes of endurance activity, and 5-10 minutes of cool-down, 3-5 days a week. Eventually the person can work up to 30 minutes of intense endurance activity, 5 days a week.

Recent research has found that overuse injuries are common when a certain threshold of heavy work is surpassed without appropriate gradual progression. Dr. Ken Cooper (1986) has recently commented "Those who are jogging more than 15 miles a week are doing it for some other reason than the health of it." People who aerobic dance more than 4 hours a week can produce niggling injuries, some of them serious enough to make the participant lay off activity to heal (Conn, Williams, & Wallace, 1982).

Regularity without injury gives much more lasting physiological benefits than irregularity with time off for healing overuse injuries.

Workout frequency also depends upon the activity. Jogging, bicycling, swimming, or aerobic dance 3 or 4 days a week is intense enough to produce good fitness benefits and should not be done more than 5 days a week. Walking, on the other hand, is less intense and therefore, should be done more frequently—at least 5 or 6 days a week, but if done 7 days a week, one or two of those days should be less intense.

When dealing with chronic disease patients in the first 8-10 weeks after discharge, or when they are severely deconditioned, it is the usual program to have them exercise for short periods of time (10-15 minutes) as often as two times a day, 7 days a week. In this manner, the exercise is performed at such a low intensity that frequency becomes the training mechanism. With patients who are progressing toward returning to work, try to match or mimic the activities of their occupations. For example, we brought cinder blocks into the exercise laboratory in the last week of a bricklayer's program, in order to check his heart rate, blood pressure, and rhythms while he did what he would be doing when he returned to work the next week.

Highly Trained or Superior Athlete

A question you might ask is, "Will training at AT make a person more fit than would the average program designed for the general fitness program person?" Yes, it will, eventually. For the non-exerciser who begins a program, the most significant improvement in fitness physiological parameters occurs in the first 8-12 weeks of physical activity. Frequency and length of workout also play a part in producing fitness gains. The superior athlete once also started as a beginner, but progressed until he worked regularly at AT, 5-6 days a week on a regular program that included strength, flexibility speed work, warm up and cool down and was specific to the activity (i.e., if he was a swimmer, he swam; if he was a skiier, he skied, etc.). The workouts that the superior athlete goes through are all-encompassing and take up as much time in a day as a full time job. There are penalties for this that have already been mentioned. These athletes constantly have injuries such as shin splints, tendinitis, pulled groin muscles, over-use problems and they are constantly nursing some part of their anatomy. That is a price they pay for being superior athletes and pursuing the limelight of the winners' circle. Training at AT will produce athletes rather than recreational and health exercisers. The exercise prescription becomes more intense the greater the level of achievement desired. The prescription increases not only the intensity but also the length of each bout of exercise and the frequency.

Concluding Remarks to Section II

This is the point where a magic formula should somehow appear, providing the secret for an exercise prescription for people of all shapes, sizes, degrees of condition, and pathologies. As you have become aware, though, each person who comes to you is unique in background, genetic structure, degree of conditioning, and many other aspects. Because of all of the differences among people, each person requires special attention. Herein lie several of the ''secrets'' of adherence to exercise. Paying special attention to the components of the unique Rx you give the participant individualizes the program and creates a desire in the participant to make it his own. Interview the person and spend time to individualize the Rx, tailoring all the parts to meet his or her needs as well as desires. You could change a life for a lifetime.

Improvisation

You might wonder what the section title ''Improvisation'' is doing in a chapter on exercise prescription. There are times when the person asking for a prescription does not meet either anatomical or functional norms. Essentially, exercise is a possibility for almost everyone, but it is a matter of degree and modality.

Musculoskeletal Disorders

These include multiple sclerosis (MS), polio, stroke, cerebral palsy, Guillain-Barre syndrome, and many others. There are several questions to be asked in reference to exercise programming with musculoskeletal problems: (a) Why do you want to exercise the person? (b) What do you hope to accomplish? (c) What is the best modality to use in prescribing exercise?

At La Crosse we have had patients with each of the above diseases and have been able to provide each patient with a successful program within the regular program, having them exercise at the same time as the other participants. There were several reasons why we worked so hard to incorporate these people into our program. Socialization and group interaction had a pronounced effect on their levels of depression and feelings of well-being. Also it appeared that in several instances, especially the Guillain-Barre syndrome and stroke victims, the patients made significant strides in recovery of strength and coordination; with the others, in some cases, disease progression seemed significantly slowed.

For most of these patients, the swimming pool afforded the best modality. Usually MS is adversely affected by warm water; however, in the case of one particular MS patient, the water felt good. The stroke victim exercised on a bicycle ergometer in the workout area where all the others were walking, jogging, or also riding bicycles. He had a deficiency on his left side that toe clips on the bicycle aided. His right leg carried his left leg through its part of the pedaling cycle. A woman with a progressive spinal disease causing increasing paralysis of the lower extremeties was able to work her arms for strength on a rehab trainer arm ergometer; then she was lowered with a Hoyer lift into the pool for a swimming program.

Skeletal Problems

Arthritis, amputation, joint replacement, and locked joints present unique problems. Once again, analyzing the problem allows the selection of an appropriate modality. For a man whose right knee and hip had been replaced, walking was not a recommended mode of exercise. Therefore, we utilized bicycle riding to warm up his extremities and provide a 10-15 minute program segment, then had him swim for the rest of his program.

Because of the design of today's prosthetic devices, sometimes it is hard to identify a person who has had a leg amputed. We recently had such a person in our Phase II program. I had not been present for his intake exam. Watching him walk on the treadmill, I noticed a bit of a limp, and I asked him if he had a sore foot. He replied that he didn't feel a thing in that leg from the midthigh down and rapped rather soundly on a chunk of wood. (Later he got what he called his "sport model" and had no limp at all.)

For arthritis patients, swimming is excellent, especially if the pool is warm. It is good to do a range-of-motion program after swimming therapy. By that time, there is a relaxation of the affected area; range of motion is increased without pain. Several of our patients have been able to reduce the amount of pain medication taken each day as they progressed in swimming programs.

Often, stress is added to diseases or anatomical problems by improper biomechanics. We make sure to teach people how to bend over, lift and carry, rise up from a lying position, stand up from a sitting position, and get out of chairs that are deep. Usually there is more weight loss, increased endurance capacity, and decrease in strength loss with these people than occurs when disease victims maintain sedentary lifestyles.

Conclusions

As you can see, the requirements for writing an exercise prescription are many. Knowledge of the disease, medications, side effects of medications, anatomical and physiological responses, and a myriad of other things is only part of the process. The patient's needs and desires become a major consideration. It is wise for you to consider all of the many areas that have been covered here and to continue to read current journals. When in doubt as to what, when, and how to prescribe, seek advice from the physician, the literature, and the experts. Exercise prescription is an exacting science, individualized for the specific person. However, because of ever-changing interventions, medications, and studies, exercise prescription is not an *exact* science—and each patient can be an exception to nearly any rule which might be written.

Appendix A

These background questions are designed to elicit information about a person's activity preferences and degree of participation in those activities. They also provide background information that will be useful when you are formulating the exercise prescription.

Background Questions for Exercise Prescription

1. What kinds of activities did you do as a child?
   a. Team sports?
   b. Individual sports?
   c. Did your family hunt, fish, hike, or camp?
   d. Did you bicycle, roller-skate, row, or swim?
   e. What did you like to do for activity when there was no one else to play with?
   f. Were there special winter activities that you liked?
2. Did you play competitive sports while growing up?
   a. Little league?
   b. Junior high sports?
   c. Club sports?
   d. High school varsity athletics?
3. Did you continue with specific activities after high school?
   a. Individual or team?
   b. How would you describe your activities since high school?
      1) Weekend only.
      2) Occasional spurts of high activity.
      3) Regular exercise (at least 3 days per week, 20-plus minutes per day).

   c. How would you describe your activities over the last year?
     1) Work- and house upkeep-related only.
     2) Spasmodic at best.
     3) Regular.

4. Are you comfortable doing, and do you like to do, the following?
   a. Walking for at least 20 minutes without stopping?
   b. Bicycling for at least 20-30 minutes continuously?
   c. Swimming in a pool or lake in water over your head?
   d. Aerobic dance, jazzercise, or aerobic exercise?
   e. Weight lifting?
   f. Rowing?
   g. Other?

Appendix B

For most people, physical activity should not pose any problem or hazard. PAR-Q has been designed to identify the small number of adults for whom physical activity might be inappropriate or who should have medical advice concerning the type of activity most suitable for them.

Physical Activity Readiness Questionnaire

1. Has your doctor ever said you have heart trouble?
2. Do you frequently suffer from pains in your chest?
3. Do you often feel faint or have spells of severe dizziness?
4. Has a doctor ever told you that you have a bone or joint problem, such as arthritis, that has been aggravated by exercise, or might be made worse with exercise?
5. Is there a good physical reason not mentioned here why you should not follow an activity program even if you want to?
6. Are you over 65 and not accustomed to vigorous exercise?

If a person answers yes to any question, vigorous exercise or exercise testing should be postponed. Medical clearance may be necessary.

References

Abbott, J.A., Hirschfield, D.S., Kunkel, F.W., et al. (1977). Graded exercise testing in patients with sinus node dysfunction. *American Journal of Medicine, 62,* 330.

American College of Sports Medicine. (1986). *Guidelines for exercise testing and prescription*. Philadelphia: Lea & Febiger.

Anderson, R. (1987). Upper body exercise. In L.K. Hall & G.C. Meyer (Eds.), *Exercise testing, exercise prescription and rehabilitation*, Champaign, IL: Human Kinetics.

Borg, G. (1970). Perceived exertion as an indicator of somatic stress. *Scandinavian Journal of Rehabilitative Medicine*, **2**, 92.

Bruce, R.A. (1973). Principles of exercise testing. In J.P. Naughton & H.K. Hellerstein (Eds.), *Exercise testing and exercise training in coronary heart disease*. New York: Academic Pres.

Conn, E., Williams, R.S., & Wallace, A.G. (1982). Exercise responses before and after physical conditioning in patients with severely depressed left ventricular function. *American Journal of Cardiology*, **49**, 296.

Cooper, K. (1986, June). Comments on fitness. *USA Today*, p. 4-D.

Ellestad, M.H. (1980). *Stress testing* (2nd ed.). Philadelphia: F.A. Davis.

Ellestad, M.H., & Wan, M.K.C. (1975). Predictive implications of stress testing, follow-up of 2700 subjects after maximal treadmill stress testing. *Circulation*, **51**, 363.

Fabian, J., Stolz, I., Janota, M., & Rohac, J. (1975). Reproducibility of exercise tests in patients with symptomatic ischemic heart disease. *British Heart Journal*, **37**, 785.

Fagin, E.T., Wayne, V.S., & McConachy, D.L. (1984). Serious ventricular arrhythmias in cardiac rehabilitation programs. *Medical Journal of Australia*, **57**, 920.

Franklin, B.A., Hellerstein, H.K., Gordon, S., & Timmis, G.C. (1986). Exercise prescription for the myocardial infarction patient. *Journal of Cardiopulmonary Rehabilitation*, **6**(2), 62-81.

Hall, L.K. (1987). Protocols. In L.K. Hall & G.C. Meyer (Eds.), *Exercise prescription, exercise testing and rehabilitation*. Champaign, IL: Human Kinetics.

Haskell, W.L., & Wenger, N.K. (1974, January). *The exercise prescription*. Network for Continuing Medical Education.

Hellerstein, H.K. (1973). *Principles of exercise prescription. Exercise testing and exercise training in coronary heart disease*. Philadelphia: Academic Press.

Hinkle, L.E., Carver, S.T., & Plankun, A. (1972). Slow heart rates and increased risk of cardiac death in middle-aged men. *Archives of Internal Medicine*, **129**, 732.

Jose, A.D., & Taylor, R.R. (1969). Autonomic blockade by propranolol and atropine to study intrinsic myocardial function in man. *Journal of Clinical Investigations*, **48**, 2019.

Karvonen, M., Kentala, K., & Mustala, O. (1957). The effects of training on heart rate: A longitudinal study. *Annales Medicinae Experimentalis et Biologieae Fenniae*, **35**, 307.

Lampman, R.M., Steward, J.R., Collins, J.A., & Thrall, J.H. (1982). Exercise training soon after left ventricular aneurysmectomy and endocardial resection. *Journal of Cardiac Rehabilitation, 2*, 134.

LeTac, B., Cribier, A., & Desplanches, J.F. (1977). A study of left ventricular function in coronary patients before and after physical training. *Circulation, 56*, 375.

McArdle, W.D., Katch, F.I., & Katch, V.L. (1981). *Exercise physiology: Energy, nutrition, and human performance*. Philadelphia: Lea & Febiger.

Meyer, G.C. (1984). The role of circuit interval and continuous conditioning in cardiac rehabilitation. In L.K. Hall, G.C. Meyer, & H.K. Hellerstein (Eds.), *Cardiac rehabilitation: Exercise testing and prescription* (pp. 193-204). Jamaica, NY: S.P. Medical.

Morris, S.N., & McHenry, P.L. (1977). The incidence and significance of exercise-induced hypotension. *American Journal of Cardiology, 39*, 289.

PAR-Q Validation Report Modified Version. (1985, June). British Columbia Canada: Department of Health.

Porter, G. (1984). General concepts and a specific approach to phase II exercise programming. In L.K. Hall, G.C. Meyer, & H.K. Hellerstein (Eds.), *Cardiac Rehabilitation: Exercise testing and prescription* (pp. 205-222). Jamaica, NY: S.P. Medical.

Rijneke, R.D. (1980). Clinical significance of upsloping S-T segments in exercise electrocardiography. *Circulation, 61*, 671.

Rozanski, J.J., Dimich, I., Steinfeld, L., & Kupersmith, J. (1979). Maximal exercise stress testing in evaluation of arrhythmias in children: Results and reproducibility. *American Journal of Cardiology, 43*, 951.

Sheps, D.S., et al. (1979). Exercise-induced increase in diastolic pressure: Indicator of severe coronary artery disease. *American Journal of Cardiology, 43*, 708.

Superko, H.R. (1983). Effects of cardiac rehabilitation in permanently paced patients with third-degree heart block. *Journal of Cardiac Rehabilitation, 3*, 561.

Wenger, N.K., & Hellerstein, H.K. (1984). *Rehabilitation of the coronary patient* (2nd ed.). New York: Wiley Medical.

Chapter 7

Body Fuel Metabolism and Diabetes

James W. Terman

Diabetes mellitus is a cluster of diseases that cause profound disturbances in the body's fuel metabolism. These diseases create a chain reaction of biochemical abnormalities by damaging a strategic step in the body's internal ecology. Over time, they lead to serious structural and functional impairments.

All living things require energy to carry out the activities of life. Higher animals, for example, use energy for all active functions, such as muscular contraction, manufacture of cellular substances, maintenance of membrane electrical charge, and production of glandular secretions. The sun is the original source of this energy. Solar energy is stored in the form of complex organic molecules in plants and animals that we use for food. This energy could be released by the process of combustion; however, such a sudden burst of heat would be intolerable to biologic tissues. Instead, organisms have evolved complex mechanisms for breaking the combustion process down into scores of steps of chemical oxidation, releasing the energy stored in food into small, safe, usable packets. The highlights of this physiological process and the alterations of it caused by diabetes are the subjects of this presentation. The purpose of this review is to lay a partial foundation for the understanding of the presentations to follow.

Normal Energy Metabolism

Higher animals eat to obtain their fuel. In mammals, before entering into the processes of energy metabolism within body tissues, the constituents of this fuel (food) must be reorganized by digestive processes from the form contained in the foodstuff into a chemical form that can be absorbed by the intestine and used by body cells. Digestion, the details of which

145

are beyond the scope of this discussion, converts starches into simple sugars such as glucose, proteins into amino acids, and fats into fatty acids and glycerol. These are the starting points for the body's energy metabolism. The focus of this discussion will concern carbohydrate metabolism, in particular that of glucose, for it is the major fuel source of most cells.

The simple reaction that the body accomplishes in combustion of glucose is

$$C_6 H_{12} O_6 + 6O_2 \rightarrow 6CO_2 + 6H_2O + \text{energy}.$$

However, the organism must accomplish this extraction of energy from its fuel while observing some constraints, which include:

1. The fuel (glucose) must be transported from the gut to distant tissues.
2. The organism must adapt to marked variability in its fuel supply, being able to function in time of plenty and subsist for periods of fasting. Thus, storage or reservoir compartments are needed to supply short-term, intermediate, and long-term energy demands.
3. It is impractical for all tissues to have all energy conversion and storage functions within their own boundaries. The problems of bulk alone would interfere with functions of specialized tissues such as muscle and brain. Thus, a central "processing area" (liver) has evolved. This, in turn, adds to the complexities of transportation. However, tissues needing temporary fuel storage for bursts of activity have this capability (such as from muscle glycogen).
4. The complex requirements of supply, storage, interconversion, and delivery of molecules and energy must be signaled by an even more sophisticated control system that usually runs automatically in order to free the organism for other life tasks. However, it still must be somewhat responsive to the cognitive activity of the brain. For example, one must be able to run from the dinner table if a fire starts in the kitchen.
5. In order to maintain chemical balance within body cells and fluids, counterregulatory mechanisms must be available to moderate physiological processes. For example, if something causes the blood glucose level to drop, counterforce must be activated to raise the glucose level to normal.
6. As mentioned earlier, simple combustion of glucose within cells would be destructive. Within cell confines, energy must be siphoned off in small steps.
7. Lastly for this discussion, most systems should have fallback systems in case of primary malfunction. Furthermore, many body organs must serve more than one function. For example, adipose

tissue is first a long-term energy warehouse; it also serves as insulation, padding, and cosmetic infrastructure.

Glucose Pathways

Glucose is actively transported across the intestine into the portal vein blood and to the liver. It also can pass into the main bloodstream, joining the circulating blood. In order to be metabolized or stored, glucose must enter cells. Without insulin, the amount that can diffuse into body cells, except those of the brain and liver, is too little to provide energy. The hormone insulin allows rapid movement of glucose into cells. As a matter of fact, it can be said that the rate of glucose metabolism in the body is for most purposes controlled by the *amount of insulin produced* by the pancreas. Thus, at this point let us leave the discussion of glucose temporarily to consider insulin.

Insulin

The pancreas is a multifunctioning organ, one part of which secretes digestive juices directly into drainage ducts headed for the duodenum. The islets of Langerhans, the truly endocrine parts of the pancreas, secrete hormones directly into the bloodstream. There are three major types of islet cells—alpha, beta, and delta—which can be distinguished when stained and examined under a microscope. Each secretes a different hormone: Beta cells produce insulin, alpha cells produce glucagon, and delta cells secrete somatostatin.

Insulin is a protein containing 51 amino acids in two chains, A and B, connected by disulfide bonds (see Figure 1). There are small, but significant, differences in the amino acids of insulin produced by humans, hogs, and cattle. Until recently, most commercial insulin preparations were made from a combination of beef and pork sources. Recently, humanlike insulin has been manufactured by recombinant gene technology.

Glucose is the chief signal for insulin synthesis. It is manufactured first in a complex, but inactive, form called proinsulin, in which a connecting (c-) peptide is present to promote correct alignment of the two main parts of the insulin molecule. Within the islet cell, the connecting peptide is removed; cellular granules containing mature insulin reach the cell surface and are secreted into the bloodstream.

The pancreas responds very swiftly to the first hint of a rise in blood sugar. Other triggers that cause insulin release are amino acids, fatty acids, acetylcholine, certain intestinal hormones, and beta adrenergic catecholamines. Insulin release is strongly affected by the prevailing glucose level. One can understand that various drugs and phenomena that modify these

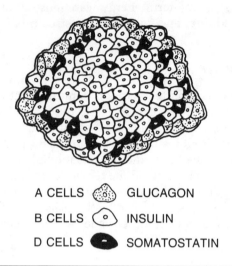

A CELLS GLUCAGON

B CELLS INSULIN

D CELLS SOMATOSTATIN

Figure 1 There are three major types of Islet of Langerhans cells: alpha, beta, and delta.

stimulators and inhibitors can, in turn, have their effect on insulin release and glucose level.

Insulin has several effects, the overall impact of which is to accomplish all the tasks necessary to an organism that has recently been fed. In the liver it promotes passage of glucose into cells, converts glucose into the storage form of glycogen, or promotes glucose breakdown for energy. Insulin triggers these actions in the liver by modulating the effect of enzymes. Insulin also promotes the conversion of glucose into fatty acids.

In muscles, the effects of insulin are more specialized. Between meals the resting muscle gets by on fatty acids and uses very little glucose. Because of increased capillary surface area during heavy exercise, glucose is highly permeable into muscle cells even without much insulin effect. For a period of time following a large meal, when both blood glucose and insulin levels are high, there is a rapid transport of glucose into the muscle cells enabling them to use carbohydrates in preference to fatty acids. If the muscles are not working in the postprandial state, much of the glucose is stored in the form of muscle glycogen as an energy source for later use. However, muscle glycogen cannot be reconverted into glucose for release into the bloodstream; it must be used within muscle cells.

The principal effect of insulin elsewhere in the body is to promote the transport of glucose through cell membranes. Without insulin, glucose cannot pass through cell membrane pores, but must be transported slowly through the fatty portion of the membrane. The first action of insulin is to bind to the outer membrane of the target cell at specific receptors, which are complex proteins that each have a unique shape fitting the insulin molecule, residing in the membrane of the cell. Thus, the cell recognizes the presence of insulin and also initiates a series of intracellular events when insulin attaches. It is currently theorized that a second intracellular "messenger compound" is activated. This second messenger activates intracellular enzymes and protein synthesis, which in turn create the characteristic insulin effects and also "open the door" to the passage of glucose into the cell (see Figure 2). A great deal of research is presently being done on the role of insulin receptors and second messengers in normal organisms, as well as in those with diabetes. Insulin receptors are steadily changing entities with half-lives of a few hours. Their presence is very susceptible to regulation by the basal insulin level, diet, hormones, and drugs.

Insulin has significant effect on other metabolic processes. For example, insulin triggers reactions that increase fat storage in adipose tissue. It promotes fatty acid synthesis in the liver and fat cells, which dovetails with the action of insulin in increasing the transport of glucose into liver cells. It inhibits an important enzyme (hormone-sensitive lipase) that causes the breakdown of triglycerides in fat cells. The net effect is to reduce the release of fatty acids into circulating blood. Finally, insulin promotes glucose transport into fat cells as with other body tissues.

Insulin causes active transport of many amino acids into cells, increases the formation of new intracellular proteins by boosting messenger RNA, increases the rate of formation of DNA, obstructs the breakdown of proteins, and retards the transformation of amino acids into glucose in the liver. Thus, the effect of insulin after a meal is to promote protein synthesis and storage, again consistent with its role as a hormone of the fed state.

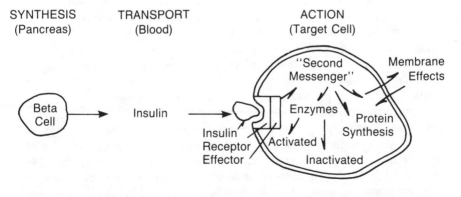

Figure 2 The second messenger activates intracellular enzymes and protein synthesis, which create the characteristic effects and also "open the door" to passage of glucose into the cell.

Taken from the point of view of the level of sugar in the bloodstream, it is thus clear that the net effect of insulin is to reduce blood sugar, ideally from high to normal levels. The body has evolved to recognize situations in which the blood sugar level declines too far, and has at its command a variety of counterregulatory mechanisms. The reason for such careful maintaining of a narrow range of blood sugar (glucose homeostasis) is that brain cells, the support and protection of which are accorded the highest priority of body processes, are totally dependent on a steady supply of glucose—their only source of energy. Insulin is not required for the entry of glucose into brain cells, but if the cells are deprived of glucose for even a brief period, severe brain dysfunction and even permanent damage can result. Counterregulatory mechanisms respond to hypoglycemia very swiftly. The most prominent of these is the other islet hormone, glucagon. We will thus continue our digression from the glucose story to consider these counterregulatory mechanisms.

Glucose Counterregulation: Glucagon et al.

Glucagon is a relatively small protein of 29 amino acids produced by the alpha cells of the islet. It is quite potent. Its production is regulated by the blood glucose concentration in a fashion opposite to that of insulin: A decrease in blood glucose increases glucagon secretion even when the blood glucose falls merely to 70 milligrams percent. Exercise can trigger glucagon secretion by lowering blood sugar. When a very high protein meal is consumed, amino acids enhance insulin secretion and would ordinarily tend to decrease blood glucose. A mechanism is present, however, for the same amino acids to cause the release of glucagon, which nullifies insulin action in this instance.

The most significant and rapid effect of glucagon is to trigger a multistep process in the liver that converts glycogen to glucose-1-phosphate, which is in turn dephosphorylated and released into the bloodstream. In this cascade of reactions, a second intracellular messenger, adenyl cyclase, is activated, which then leads to an ever-amplifying sequence of enzyme actions that eventually unlock glucose from its polymer glycogen. Glucagon can also initiate the process of gluconeogenesis, in which amino acids, lactate, and pyruvate are converted into glucose.

Epinephrine, a hormone secreted by the central medulla of the adrenal gland and by the sympathetic nervous system, enters the circulation at times of stress or falling blood presssure. It has many effects on the heart and circulation; in fuel metabolism it has an effect like that of glucagon in causing liver glycogenolysis. Indeed, many of the early symtoms of hypoglycemia are actually spillover effects of epinephrine on other systems in the body.

A brief mention should be made of the more recently discovered hormone-like agent somatostatin. This is illustrated in Figure 3. It is

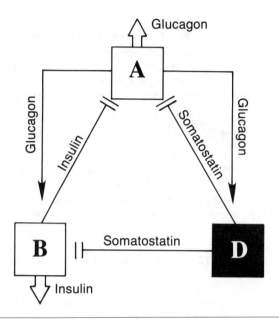

Figure 3   Somatostatin plays a key role in the interaction of islet hormones.

secreted by the delta cells of the islets and appears to have a restraining effect on the secretion of both insulin and glucagon, inhibitory effects on the absorption of nutrients from the gut, and negative effects on certain pituitary hormones. Its role is not totally clear, but it has multiple effects on various parts of the body; it seems to function as a restrainer or negative modulator of the primary regulatory mechanisms of glucose level and helps maintain very sophisticated control of blood sugar. Other substances that have an effect on these activities, but won't be considered here, include growth hormone, beta endorphins, cortisol, sex hormones, and gastrointestinal hormones. Some of these effects do become important in the analysis of long-standing, poorly controlled diabetes mellitus.

The foregoing side trip into hormones and other mechanisms that regulate glucose control gives an indication of the survival importance of glucose homeostasis. The mechanisms allow the organisms that own them to adapt to and survive a very wide variety of environmental circumstances.

Glucose Within Body Cells

Resuming the tour that glucose takes through the body, we have up to this point followed it across an insulin-guided traverse of a cell membrane.

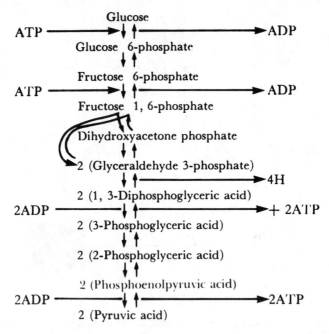

Net reaction:

Glucose + 2ADP + 2PO$_4$$^{---}$ ⟶ 2 Pyruvic acid + 2ATP + 4H

Figure 4   The separate phases of glycolysis. *Note.* From *Textbook of Medical Physiology* (6th ed.) (p. 843) by A.C. Guyton, 1981, Philadelphia: W.B. Saunders. Copyright 1981 by W.B. Saunders Company. Reprinted by permission.

If it is not to be stored, glucose is broken down and oxidized for energy in a complex process that can be considered in separate phases (see Figure 4; Guyton, 1981). The first phase is called glycolysis, during which the six-carbon glucose atom is disassembled into two three-carbon molecules of pyruvic acid. It takes 10 sequential steps of chemical reactions to do this. Use is made of the attachment of phosphate radicals, the bonding processes of which can potentially make available a great deal of energy. A succession of different enzymes is required to catalyze each step of the process. Not a lot of energy is released at this time. At the end of the glycolytic phase, however, enough energy is available to form a certain amount of an energy-carrying intermediate molecule, adenosine triphosphate (ATP).

ATP—Energy Currency

ATP is worthy of special mention. This is a highly changeable chemical compound made up of a nucleic acid, adenine, joined to a five-carbon

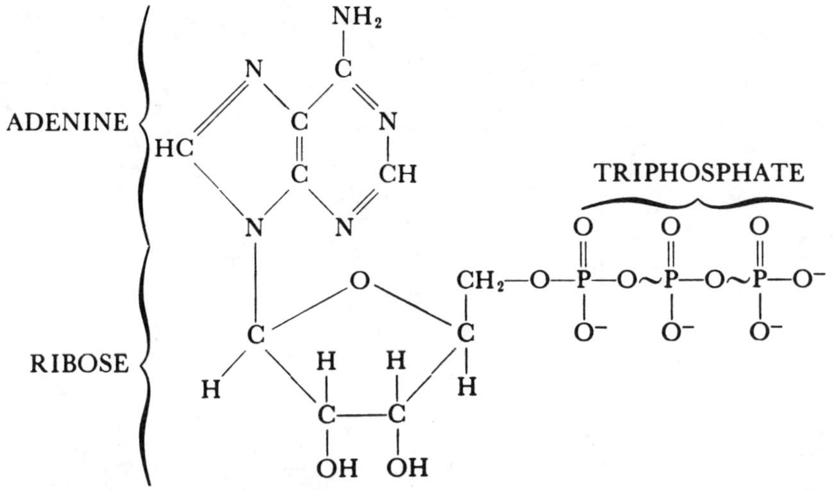

Figure 5   The highest level of energy conversion is ATP. *Note.* From *Textbook of Medical Physiology* (6th ed.) (p. 839) by A.C. Guyton, 1981, Philadelphia: W.B. Saunders. Copyright 1981 by W.B. Saunders Company. Reprinted by permission.

sugar, ribose, which is in turn hooked to one, two, or three phosphate radicals (PO_4). The bondings between successive phosphate portions carry energy. The highest energy level version is ATP (see Figure 5; Guyton, 1981). Subtracting one phosphate releases energy and a lower power molecule, adenosine disphosphate (ADP); an even lower energy product results when the number two phosphate is cleaved off, yielding adenosine monophosphate (AMP). The reactions between ADP, ATP, and energy are found in virtually every energy-releasing chemical step of the body. Approximately 8,000 calories of energy are transferred for each mole (gram-molecular weight) of ATP. When a body chemical reaction releases energy, ADP absorbs it with phosphate to become ATP; ATP then can be transported to other sites, passing along the energy and becoming ADP once again; then the ADP can be used to re-form ATP. At best, there is always a steady supply of this agent and, because it is located in virtually all areas of the cell, a parallel has been drawn between its role in energy transfer to that of money in the economic system. There are other compounds in tissues that use high energy phosphate bonds in energy exchange—for example, creatine phosphate in muscle—but the ATP system is the principal energy carrier in all body tissues.

Returning to glucose metabolism, we have discussed the fact that the first phase of it, glycolysis, generates some ATP during the conversion to pyruvic acid. This is only a small portion of the potential energy that could be extracted from the glucose molecule; however, the glycolysis phase does have the advantage of not requiring oxygen. It is the source

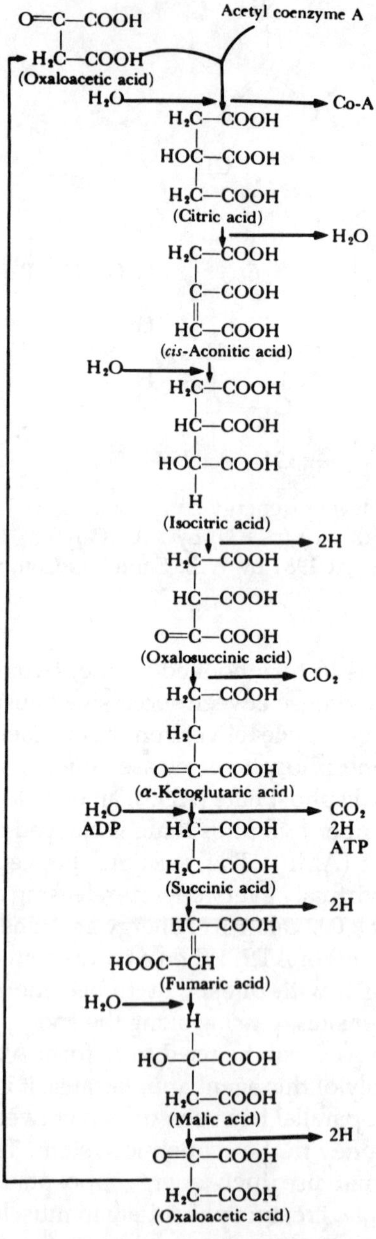

Figure 6 This sequence of chemical reactions is called the Krebs, citric acid, cycle. From *Textbook of Medical Physiology* (6th ed.) (p. 843) by A.C. Guyton, 1981, Philadelphia: W.B. Saunders. Copyright 1981 by W.B. Saunders Company. Reprinted by permission.

of energy during anaerobic exercise, for example. The second phase, occurring in intracellular structures called mitochondria, consists of a sequence of chemical reactions called the citric acid (Krebs) cycle. Figure 6 illustrates this cycle (Guyton, 1981). It is preceded by the conversion of pyruvic acid into a two-carbon acetyl molecule by conjunction with a carrier molecule known as coenzyme A(CoA). Acetyl CoA then enters the Krebs cycle, a sequence of approximately nine major steps out of which carbon dioxide, water, energy in the form of ATP, and the original coenzyme A are generated (or regenerated).

An alternative system for oxidizing glucose is through the pentose shunt (also known as the hexose monophosphate shunt), which can account for as much as 30% of the glucose breakdown in the liver and in fat cells. It serves as a backup system in case there is an abnormality of the Krebs cycle. Glucose phosphate is slowly oxidized to a five-carbon sugar, ribulose, with release of energy to ATP.

Free hydrogen atoms, which also are a source of energy, are another by-product of glycolysis, the Krebs cycle, and the pentose shunt. These atoms are stored temporarily on a complex derivative of the vitamin niacin, nicotine adenine dinucleotide (NAD). Looking back on all the glucose breakdown cycles we have discussed, in total they release only a small portion of the potential energy available in the original glucose molecule. In actuality, about 90% of the possible final ATP is formed by subsequent oxidation of the hydrogen atoms stored on NAD (NADH) into water; indeed, it has been said that the principal function of all of these earlier stages is to make the hydrogen of the glucose molecule available in a form that can be utilized for oxidation. The subsequent oxidation of hydrogen is accomplished by a series of small reactions that change the hydrogen atoms into charged hydrogen ions and free electrons; the latter are used to change the dissolved oxygen of cell fluids into hydroxyl ions. Then the hydrogen and hydroxyl ions combine to form water, during which process a tremendous quantity of energy is released into more ATP. During these changes, the electrons released are handed through a metabolic "bucket brigade" of chemicals attached to the mitochondria. These chemicals include flavoproteins, cytochromes, and other molecules that finally allow the conversion of ADP into ATP.

For each molecule of glucose that enters the complete energy metabolism cycles of cells, there are 2 molecules of ATP generated during glycolysis, 2 molecules of ATP during the citric acid cycle, up to 30 ATP molecules during the hydrogen transfer reactions, plus 4 more from other areas of the scheme, yielding a maximum of 38 ATP molecules for each molecule of glucose that is totally broken down into carbon dioxide and water. The overall maximum efficiency of energy transfer is about 44%, the remaining 56% being used up in heat.

Other Energy Sources

It is evident that fats and proteins can also become energy sources. A brief mention of fat oxidation follows. The basic unit of fat is the triglyceride molecule, made up of the three-carbon alcohol glycerol unified with three long chain fatty acids. Almost all cells, except for those of the brain, can use fatty acids, in addition to glucose for energy. The fatty acid molecule, after being split off from glycerol, is degraded by mitochodria, with sequential release of two carbon acetyl CoA molecules, which can enter into the citric acid cycle. This process potentially provides a great deal more energy per molecule of fatty acid than does glucose. For example, stearic acid can be converted into 146 molecules of ATP. Unfortunately for diabetes, a large part of this metabolism occurs in the liver; there much of the acteyl CoA can condense to form acetoacetic acid, which is then converted into beta-hydroxybutyric acid. A small amount of free acetone is produced; these are the "ketone bodies," which then diffuse through the liver into blood and peripheral tissues. During starvation and diabetic ketoacidosis, a large quantity builds up and contributes to the pathologies of those states.

Summary

In summary, we have followed a molecule of glucose through a complex and zigzag tour through the body metabolism, with side excursions into related mechanisms. As complex as it may seem, this description has been highly simplified for the purposes of this discussion. One may look back through these mechanisms and judge for oneself whether they satisfy the seven demands, enumerated earlier, that free-living animals must observe. These mechanisms do provide the adaptability, sophisticated control of regulation, homeostasis, controlled energy release, and reserve pathways that are required. The next part of this chapter will concern the alterations in these mechanisms produced during the disease state of diabetes mellitus.

Biochemistry of Diabetes

Now that we have explored the process of normal energy metabolism, it will be easier to enter into a discussion of how diabetes mellitus causes deviations from this process. I will describe these deviations and some of their effects in the following pages.

Classification of Diabetes Mellitus

It is currently believed that diabetes is a syndrome of various causes, characterized by a partial or a complete inadequacy of either production, delivery, or use of insulin during the fuel metabolism process. For the purposes of this discussion, we will not consider the secondary forms of diabetes associated with chronic pancreatic disease, hormone excess, drug effects, or certain rare genetic syndromes. Instead, we will deal with Type I diabetes (insulin-dependent diabetes mellitus: IDDM) and Type II diabetes mellitus (non-insulin-dependent: NIDDM). Type I used to be known as *juvenile* or *brittle* diabetes, even though it can start in maturity; Type II used to be thought of as *adult onset* diabetes, even though it can develop in the relatively young. The Type I diabetic is distinguished by absolute dependence on external injection of insulin to prevent ketosis and preserve life (even though there may be transient non-insulin-dependent phases of the disease's evolution). The Type II diabetic, even though prescribed insulin, is not completely dependent on exogenous insulin and in its absence does not develop ketoacidosis. Although roughly 80% of Type II diabetics are obese, there is a nonobese subcategory.

No firm answers are available to describe each type's cause. Current evidence, however, suggests that Type I diabetes is more apt to occur sporadically, particularly in persons with certain forms of tissue antigens (HLA). This form of diabetes is more apt to appear following certain viral infections. Recent research focuses on virus-triggered immunologic damage to beta cells. Type II diabetes has a considerable hereditary component. Unfortunately, the type of intrinsic factors that eventually lead to overt Type II diabetes have not been identified. Type II diabetes is usually preceded by a subclinical phase of sluggish production of insulin after glucose ingestion and may become overt in periods of stress, pregnancy, medication use, and so on. Most commonly it appears in an obese person growing older.

When fully developed, diabetes, as can be reasoned from the first section of this presentation, is characterized by chronic abnormalities of the metabolism not only of carbohydrates, but also of fat and protein. Furthermore, chronic diabetes brings on eventual disorders of the structure and function of blood vessels and of tissues that depend on their vasculature. The principal abnormalities of Type I diabetes are related to complete insulin deficiency; the abnormalities most often seen in Type II diabetes are those of delayed or uncoordinated release of endogenous insulin.

Normal and Abnormal Glucose Homeostasis

The previously described homeostatic mechanisms keep the blood glucose level in the fasting postabsorptive state between 60 and 110 milligrams per deciliter (milligrams percent). Following the ingestion of a 75-gram glucose drink, the normal blood sugar rises rapidly to a peak at 60 minutes of 120-140, and rarely above 160, milligrams percent. This peak can be seen in Figure 7 (Lilly Research Laboratories, 1980). Insulin

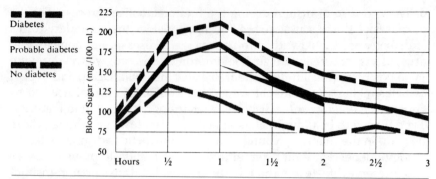

Figure 7   The blood sugar responses after oral ingestion of a 75-gram glucose load. The wedge shape denotes a borderline area. *Note.* From *Diabetes Mellitus* (8th ed.) (p. 4) by Lilly Research Laboratories, 1980, Indianapolis: Author. Copyright 1980 by Lilly Research Laboratories. Reprinted by permission.

rapidly lowers the blood sugar to the normal range by 2 hours after ingestion. The diagnosis of diabetes is made by the finding of persistently elevated blood glucose in the fasting state or postprandial blood glucose that is above a certain level and is slow to return to normal. The criteria for the diagnosis of diabetes have been the objects of years of epidemiologic research. It should be pointed out that the oral glucose tolerance test, if chosen, should be applied with attention to detail. Also, the criteria are different in special circumstances, such as starvation states, pregnancy, and old age.

Approximately half of the patients with untreated diabetes have classical symptoms, including weight loss, excessive thirst, excessive urination, excessive consumption of liquids, and excessive hunger. Other symptoms—including blurred vision, weakness, fatigue, recurrent skin infections, and yeast infections—also may be clues. In Type II diabetes, the diagnosis is sometimes made by the discovery of certain long-term complications, such as neuropathy, arteriosclerosis, or visual impairment.

Biochemical Abnormalities in Untreated Type I Diabetes

The scarred beta islet cells are unable to produce enough insulin. The glucose concentration commonly rises to 500-600 milligrams per deciliter. At the same time, there are elevated glucagon concentrations. At this stage it may be simplistically thought that the body is sensing intracellular starvation. Table 1 describes the clinical and biochemical correlates of the diabetic syndrome (Kozak, 1982). Insulin deficiency permits the breakdown of stored fat and the increased flow of free fatty acids from fat cells to the liver to serve as a substitute fuel. Excess glucagon inhibits a key entity (malonyl-coenzyme A) that normally plays a central role in blocking the use of fatty acids in the liver. Fatty acids can then be admitted to the liver cell and burned. There are other gluconeogenic pathways also activated in the liver.

A by-product of combustion of fatty acids by the liver is overproduction of two strong short chain fatty acids, beta-hydroxybutyric acid and acetoacetic acid. In the bloodstream these acids begin to consume the body's acid-base buffers. At the same time, there is produced a small amount of acetone, which is exhaled from the lungs, creating the typical aromatic odor of the ketoacidosis victim. Progressive acidosis stimulates brain respiratory control centers, increasing the rate and depth of respiration. High levels of glucose and other metabolic by-products are excreted through the kidneys. They force an accompanying water excretion that, along with respiratory losses, causes progressive dehydration. Although sodium, potassium, chloride, phosphorous, and magnesium are lost, the serum concentrations of these ions may be normal. After enough dehydration occurs, such metabolic waste products as urea and creatinine accumulate, and kidney function deteriorates. Fluid shifts cause brain swelling, and excess ketones can produce a mild narcosis. In the final state, acidosis paralyzes muscles and causes cardiac arrhythmias, dehydration causes shock, and cardiac and circulatory collapse may cause death. This catastrophic downhill course comprises the state of diabetic ketoacidosis (diabetic coma). The victim may go from the first symptoms to death within a few hours if untreated.

Treatment of this medical emergency consists of the intravenous infusion of large volumes of balanced saline solutions and the immediate institution of intravenous insulin therapy. Whereas for many years a complex scheme of individual insulin injections was used, it is most common now to treat diabetic ketoacidosis with constant drip infusion of insulin, which can be regulated rather easily because of the short half-life of insulin. The physician caring for the patient repeatedly must monitor the measurements of blood sugar, ketones, arterial acid base information, electrolytes, and urine output during the resuscitation. As recovery begins, the body shifts from fatty acid to glucose metabolism as insulin permits its entry into tissue cells. The acid burden decreases. Large volumes of potassium, phosphorous, and calcium, previously marooned in the bloodstream, can then shift into cells. The physician must be alert to this shift, because potassium must be added to the therapy at this point. Successful therapy usually takes from 6-12 hours, with 24-48 hours of regulation thereafter. Diabetic ketoacidosis is often precipitated by such stressors as infections, and these underlying factors must be searched for by the physician while treatment proceeds. Optimum care for diabetics is directed at preventing this life-threatening event; each reappearance carries further risk of an irreversible catastrophe, such as brain damage, stroke, or myocardial infarction.

Table 1   Clinical and Biochemical Correlates of the Diabetic Syndrome

Type of Metabolism	Metabolic Defects	Chemical Abnormalities	Clinical Correlates
A. Carbohydrate metabolism	1. Diminished uptake of glucose by tissues such as muscle, adipose tissue, and liver	Hyperglycemia	Polyuria Polydipsia Polyphagia Fatigue Muscle weakness Pruritus
	2. Overproduction of glucose (via glycogenolysis and gluconeogenesis) by the liver		Blurred vision Diminished mental alertness
B. Protein metabolism	1. Diminished uptake of amino acids and diminished synthesis of protein	Negative nitrogen balance Elevated levels of branched-chain amino acids Elevated blood urea nitrogen level	Loss of muscle mass Weakness
	2. Increased proteolysis	Elevated potassium level	

C. Fat metabolism		
1. Increased lipolysis	Elevated plasma fatty acids level	Loss of adipose tissue
	Elevated plasma glycerol level	Nausea and vomiting
2. Decreased lipogenesis	Elevated plasma ketones	Abdominal pain Acetone on breath
3. Increased production of triglycerides	Hypertriglyceridemia	Exudative xanthoma (skin lesions)
		Lipemia retinalis Pancreatitis (abdominal pain)
4. Decreased removal of triglycerides	Metabolic acidosis	Hyperventilation Rapid breathing

Note. From *Clinical Diabetes Mellitus* (p. 19) by G.P. Kozak, 1982, Philadelphia: W.B. Saunders. Copyright 1982 by W.B. Saunders Company. Reprinted by permission.

Long Term Treatment of the Type I Diabetic

The first priority in management of any diabetes, but particularly insulin-dependent types, is appropriate diet, the principles of which are embodied in the standard American Diabetes Association diet plans. At the present time, 50-60% of the total calories of these diets comes from carbohydrates. It is important that the majority of these carbohydrates be in complex forms, such as starches, glycogens, and cellulose. They also provide fibrous bulk, which enhances intestinal function and, according to recent evidence, may improve diabetic regulation. Sucrose and other simple sugars should be used in limited quantities, and as a part of a mixed meal or in such natural forms as fruits. In any case, they should not account for more than 10% of the total calories. Fat intake should supply no more than 30-35% of the total calories. According to current concepts, it is especially important that diabetics adhere to recommended limitations in cholesterol and saturated animal fats in order to prevent premature arteriosclerosis. The remainder of the diet should be made up of balanced proteins to supply essential amino acids.

The total caloric value of the diet is perhaps the most important thing to the diabetic, because the extremes of obesity and caloric malnutrition must be studiously avoided. The caloric intake is calculated by taking into consideration basal needs, growth needs (in children), and the needs of activity for exercise. Correction factors must be applied, based on body muscle mass, activity levels, and such special situations as pregnancy and stress. Negative correction must be applied to reduce excess weight. These principles are best translated into appropriate meal plans by experienced dieticians.

The next component of management of insulin dependent diabetes is the activity or exercise plan. Details of the response to exercise are beyond the scope here; but, broadly speaking, diabetics do best when they live on regular activity schedules that allow them to pursue the cycles of living and working but pay special attention to aerobic and fitness activities. Nutritional intake must be spaced to match different levels of energy expenditures.

Insulin dose for the Type I diabetic is the third component of management after prescribing appropriate diet and exercise level. When a therapist attempts to provide a smooth and appropriate supply of exogenous insulin, difficulties often encountered make one appreciate the sophisticated response system of the normal pancreas. Insulin has a half-life in the bloodstream of just a few minutes. Insulin cannot reach the system when given orally, because it is broken down in the intestinal tract. Thus, it must be provided by some form of deposit through the skin.

Traditionally, insulin injection has been available in short-acting (regular, semi-Lente), intermediate-acting (NPH, Lente), and long-acting forms (ultra-Lente, PZI). No one form of insulin can begin to approach the natural pancreatic response (see Table 2). Major research and develop-

Table 2   Time Curve of Insulin Action

Insulin	Initial Time (hours)	Peak Time (hours)	Duration (hours)
Rapid			
Regular	1/2-1	2-3	5-8
Semilente	1-2	4-8	12-16
Intermediate			
Globin	2-4	6-10	14-20
NPH	2-4	8-12	18-26
Lente	2-4	8-16	18-28
Long			
PZI	6-8	14-24	24-36+
Ultralente	6-8	16-24	24-36+

Note. From *Clinical Diabetes Mellitus* (p. 74). by G.P. Kozak, 1982, Philadelphia: W.B. Saunders. Copyright 1982 by W.B. Saunders Company. Reprinted by permission.

ment activity is underway to reach a technologic answer to this problem. Continuous insulin infusion by open- and closed-loop techniques are in trial and are being used by small numbers of diabetics. Multiple injection techniques have been tried. The availability of rapid estimations of blood glucose by simple finger stick methods have enhanced this capability. Some hope exists for the development of a microelectronically controlled "artificial pancreas." Other experts hope that pancreatic transplantation will provide the needed answer. The motive for this push toward a steady and responsive supply of insulin is the emerging persuasive, although not conclusive, evidence that the gap between desirable and actual blood sugars in the diabetic that exist day in and day out for years is responsible for the slowly cumulative tissue damage that builds into diabetic complications.

After the development of diabetes, there is often a "honeymoon period" in which, after initial control is established, the exogenous insulin requirement seems to decline or even disappear. Almost inevitably, with a few months this "honeymoon period" will disappear, leaving the patient entirely dependent on exogenous insulin and diabetic management. However, if meticulous control is maintained for the first few years after diagnosis, the long-term course is much freer of complications than if control is attempted after squandering this interval. With persistent hyperglycemia, though, microscopic changes ensue in basement membrane thickness, especially in blood vessels. Thereafter, blood vessel changes occur especially in the retina of the eye, the glomerulus of the kidney, and small blood vessels supplying nerve branches. These gradually progress to clinical diabetic retinopathy, renal insufficiency, and neuropathy. The exact correlation between hyperglycemia and these complications is strongly suspected but not yet proven; there may be other, as yet unevaluated, contributing factors.

Type II Diabetes Mellitus

Many features of Type I diabetes are also true of Type II diabetes. However, from the standpoint of epidemiology, and possibly of pathogenesis, the two conditions may be nearly separate diseases.

The Type II diabetic most commonly is an obese adult with a fairly strong history of mature diabetes in relatives. These patients usually have some of their own insulin, even increased amounts, but it is inefficiently produced or has inadequate effect at the tissue receptor sites. There is usually enough insulin to prevent ketoacidosis, although there can be risk of this state under certain kinds of stress. Unlike in Type I diabetes, there are no antibodies to pancreas islet cells. Type II diabetics rarely present first in ketoacidosis. Instead, they usually are detected by the incidental finding of elevated blood sugar, or they may present with mild fatigue, polyuris, polydipsia, and polyphagia. Many Type II diabetics are not diagnosed until a complication such as neuropathy appears. There is also a much stronger correlation between Type II diabetes and arteriosclerotic coronary artery disease and peripheral vascular insufficiency.

The association between obesity and Type II diabetes is well established, although not total. Obesity is probably the most frequent cause of insulin resistance. Insulin cannot influence glucose metabolism in the liver, skeletal muscle, and fatty tissue nearly as well in the obese person as in the nonobese. This type of insulin resistance in the tissues can in many cases be completely reversed through weight reduction. Furthermore, some obese Type II diabetics actually have a chronic elevation of insulin in their bloodstreams, which paradoxically seems to harm its own chances of effectiveness. Furthermore, the daily caloric intake of the obese person aggravates this very effect. Finally, there may be some degree of insulin deficiency in the Type II diabetic, especially in the nonobese minority.

As can be reasoned from the above, diet treatment is by far the most important, and nearly exclusive, form of management of the Type II diabetic. The difficult task of weight reduction, if successful, may reduce or eliminate insulin resistance, bring insulin overproduction down to normal, and "up regulate" insulin receptors on peripheral tissue cells. All of these tend to normalize blood sugar. Exercise plays an important contributing role. Under proper circumstances aerobic exercise contributes to weight loss, blocks fatty acids storage in adipose tissue, and converts atherogenic lipids to more benign forms. Exercise increases insulin sensitivity.

A lesser, and more controversial, role exists for medications and insulin in the treatment of Type II diabetes. Since many older Type II diabetics find it beyond their capability to lose weight and exercise properly, many must resort to the use of oral drugs of the sulfonylurea type to reduce blood sugar to some extent. These drugs help the symptoms of hyperglycemia in the short term. They seem to increase the pancreatic output of insulin and may increase peripheral tissue insulin receptors. Insulin itself is used in some Type II diabetics, although the effects may be disappointing, except under times of stress. As can be seen from the foregoing, many Type II diabetics already have a superabundance of insulin, and giving more will merely aggravate the negative effects on insulin receptors. Finally, it is not clear whether oral agents have some independent, adverse effect on diabetic arteriosclerotic complications.

With respect to long-term complications of the Type II diabetic, there is susceptibility to the same types of microangiopathy seen in Type I cases with chronic hyperglycemia. In addition, as mentioned, there also are more arteriosclerotic effects than with nondiabetics. Cataracts are more frequently seen in these patients, too.

The above discussion is a rapid survey intended to provide a first acquaintence or reminder of diabetes and its pertinent biochemical effects on the body. The reader is strongly urged to consult references such as those given on the reading list for more precise details.

References

Ellenburg, M., & Rifkin, H. (Eds.). (1983). *Diabetes mellitus, theory and practice* (3rd ed.). New Hyde Park, NY: Medical Examination Publishing.

Guyton, A.C. (1981). *Textbook of medical physiology* (6th ed.). Philadelphia: W.B. Saunders.

Kozak, G.P. (1982). *Clinical diabetes mellitus*. Philadelphia: W.B. Saunders.

Lilly Research Laboratories. (1980). *Diabetes mellitus* (8th ed.). Indianapolis: Author.

Rifkin, H., & Rasken, P. (Eds.). (1981). *Diabetes mellitus* (Vol. V). Bowie, MD: Brady.

Chapter 8

Evaluation and Testing of the Diabetic Patient Prior to Exercise Prescription

Barbara N. Campaigne

This chapter will describe the job of the exercise physiologist in evaluating Type I and Type II diabetic patients. When given the opportunity to evaluate a patient with diabetes who is interested in developing an exercise program, the exercise physiologist should proceed with care. A full understanding of the patient's baseline state of health, both generally and specifically related to diabetes and coronary heart disease risk, is necessary. In addition, information on other medical problems needs to be obtained before advice on exercise can be given. This chapter presents information on the screening procedures necessary for prescribing a safe, effective exercise program for patients with diabetes.

Diabetes Control and the Role of Exercise

Exercise has long been considered a component of the triad of diabetes management, along with insulin and diet. The effects of regular exercise on diabetes have been, and continue to be, subjects of intense research efforts. Table I summarizes the current findings in this area as they pertain to Type I and Type II diabetic patients. Briefly, it has been shown that regular aerobic activities can improve metabolic control in Type II patients as evidenced by decreased glycosylated hemoglobin and fasting blood glucose levels, in conjunction with decreased insulin levels (Borgardus et al., 1984; Ruderman, Ganda, & Johansen, 1979; Schneider, Amorosa, Khachadurian, & Ruderman, 1984; Trovati et al., 1984). It is generally accepted that regular exercise alone, without alteration in insulin dose or dietary intake, does not improve long-term glycemic con-

Table 1   Benefits of Regular Exercise in Patients With Diabetes

Control Variables	Type I	Type II
Glycemic control	No change in HbA$_1$	↓ HbA$_1$
Insulin sensitivity	↑ Glucose utilization	↑ Glucose utilization
Blood lipids	↓ TG	↓ TG
Lipoproteins	↑ HDL-C/TC ↓ LDL-C	
VO$_2$ Max	↑	↑
Skeletal muscle oxidative enzyme activity	↑	
Body weight		↓ (In conjunction with diet)

trol in patients with Type I diabetes (Pedersen, Beck-Nielsen, & Heding, 1980; Wallberg-Henriksson, Gunnarsson, & Henriksson, 1982; Wallberg-Henriksson, Gunnarsson, Henriksson, Ostman, & Wahren, 1984; Yki-Jarvinen, DeFranzo, & Koivisto, 1984; Zinman, Zuniga-Guajardo, & Kelly, 1984). It has been shown that regular exercise enhances tissue sensitivity to insulin both in Type I and Type II diabetes (Pederson, et al., 1980; Trovati et al., 1984; Wallberg-Henriksson et al., 1982). The insulin response to an oral glucose load has been found to improve after physical training and to be related to daily physical activity levels in those with glucose intolerance (Lingarde & Saltin, 1981; Saltin et al., 1979).

A decreased morbidity and mortality rate for those with Type I diabetes who participated in team sports in high school and college, when compared to those who did not participate, has been reported recently (LaPorte, Dorman, Tajima, Cruickshanks, Orchard, Cavender, Becker, & Drash, 1986). Those who exercised regularly were found to have a lower incidence of macrovascular complications, with the exception of retinopathy.

Coronary Heart Disease (CHD) Risk

Persons with diabetes have an approximately twofold increase in the risk for development of premature CHD, when compared to nondiabetic persons (Ganda, 1980). Abnormal lipid profiles have been implicated as one predisposing factor (Goldberg, 1981). The preventive effects of exercise on the development of CHD for nondiabetic persons has been documented recently (Blair, Goodyear, Gibbons, & Cooper, 1984; Paffenberger, Hyde, Wing, & Steinmetz, 1984). The beneficial effects of exercise on blood lipid profiles in nondiabetics have been well described (Hietanen, 1982) and may be partially attributable to the decreased CHD risk in active populations. These benefits include a decrease in plasma triglycerides (TG) and most commonly an increase in high density lipoprotein cholesterol (HDL-C). HDL-C has been shown to have a strong inverse relationship with CHD risk and is believed to act by reverse cholesterol transport (Miller, Nesteri, & Clifton-Bligh, 1976). The effects of regular exercise on lipids and lipoproteins in Type I diabetes include a decrease in TG (Larsson, Persson, Sterky, & Thoren, 1964), an increase in the HDL-C/TC ratio (Wallberg-Henriksson et al., 1982; Yki-Jarvinen et al., 1984), and a decrease in LDL-C (Campaigne et al., 1985). Other important benefits of regular exercise include increased oxygen consumption during maximal exercise (Pederson et al., 1980; Trovati et al., 1984; Wallberg-Henriksson et al., 1982; Wallberg-Henriksson et al., 1984; Yki-Jarvinen et al., 1984; Zinman et al., 1984) (thus increased fitness level) and increased skeletal muscle enzyme activity (Wallberg-Henriksson et al., 1982; Wallberg-Henriksson et al., 1984).

Weight Loss

Regular exercise has been shown to be effective as an adjunct in weight loss programs, which is important for patients with Type II diabetes (Barnard, Lattimore, Holy, Charny, & Pritikin, 1982; Nowalk, Wing, Epstein, Paternostro, & Kriska, 1985).

In summary, regular exercise has been shown to have beneficial effects on diabetes control (Type II's), insulin sensitivity, lipid profiles, cardiovascular fitness, and as an adjunct therapy to bring about lifestyle changes.

In view of the above findings, exercise has been established as a valuable component of the overall therapeutic approach to diabetes by the American Diabetes Association (1984).

Exercise Program Screening Procedures

As with any exercise program, before a safe level of exercise can be prescribed, each patient must be thoroughly evaluated. Based on the current knowledge of diabetes and its relation to CHD, the screening procedure used should be similar to that utilized with regard to CHD risk, for most of the adult population, with several requirements specific to those with diabetes.

History and Physical Examination

A history and physical examination will be necessary for newly diagnosed patients and for those who do not have accurate records available. The history should include all medications currently being taken. The physical examination should include a review of all systems in order to identify any medical problems (e.g., arthritis, asthma) that may need consideration when the individual exercise program is being developed.

Diabetes Evaluation

A glycosylated hemoglobin or hemoglobin A_1 (HbA$_1$) should be obtained. This is a means of determining long-term blood glucose control. HbA$_1$ is the portion of hemoglobin that is bound with glucose. It is present in everyone, but is usually higher in those with diabetes, depending upon their state of glycemic control. The hemoglobin A_1 reflects the average blood glucose level over the past 2-3 months (the life span of a red blood cell). Thus, it is free from transient blood glucose excursions. Along with an evaluation of diabetes control, an ophthalmascopic examination should be performed (if proliferative retinopathy is present or suspected, a detailed ophthalmascopic examination is required). A neurological examination should be completed in order to assess the presence of neuropathy. A nephrological evaluation can be made by clinical determination of the presence of microalbumin or protein in the urine. Any of these tests performed by clinics or private physicians within the previous 3 months need not be repeated. Results of any tests performed recently should be obtained from the patient's records.

Patients with Type I diabetes frequently are underweight at the time of diagnosis, whereas Type II patients often are overweight or obese. The nutritional status of the diabetic patient should be evaluated, because this may be an important variable affected by the overall therapy. For some Type I patients, weight gain may be indicated; whereas for Type II patients, weight loss often is necessary. A baseline evaluation of nutritional status, including height, weight, and anthropometric measurements (i.e., skinfolds, circumferences, diameters) or some other form of body composition assessment (i.e., hydrostatic weighing, K40), is recommended. This information should be obtained in follow-up evaluations to assess the success of the program in aiding patients to decrease body weight and maintain lean body mass concomitant to weight loss, for example, or to increase lean body mass with weight gain or weight maintenance.

Cardiovascular Evaluation

The following should be evaluated at rest: (a) blood pressure, (b) peripheral pulses, (c) bruits, (d) 12-lead electrocardiogram (ECG); in addition, a blood lipid profile (of lipids and lipoproteins) is suggested. Thorough evaluation of diabetes control may be aided by lipid profiles because lipid abnormalities are common among those with diabetes. In addition, a lipid profile aids in the overall assessment of a person's CHD risk. If a patient is over 35 years of age, or has history of suspected or documented cardiovascular disease or multiple primary CHD risk factors (i.e., smoking, hypertension, elevated blood cholesterol), a graded exercise test (GXT) should be performed. A GXT evaluation should include ECG and blood pressure monitoring throughout, in accordance with guidelines of the American College of Sports Medicine (1986). Both the diabetes evaluation and the cardiovascular evaluation should be used in developing an individualized exercise program for each patient. In addition, any other medical problems (e.g., arthritis, asthma) should be considered in developing the exercise program.

Contraindications for *strenuous* physical exercise include

- poor metabolic control (e.g., ketosis),
- active proliferative retinopathy,
- evidence of cardiovascular disease,
- microangiopathy,
- neuropathy,
- nephropathy.

Patients contraindicated to specific types of exercise (e.g., because of insensitive feet) should be carefully guided in those activities that are most appropriate (e.g., cycling or swimming).

Exercise Prescription

Every program should start with a low work load based on the person's previous level of exercise or graded exercise test results. Heart rate and, when necessary, blood pressure response should be monitored during exercise sessions. After initial evaluation each patient should be given an individualized exercise prescription, with training heart rate according to the guidelines of the American College of Sports Medicine (1986). The patient should be encouraged to remain in contact with the diabetes management group (i.e., physician, exercise physiologist, dietician, etc.). A copy of all screening results and exercise prescriptions should be mailed to the private physician. It is recommended to both the patient and private physician that the patient be reevaluated at the Diabetes Management Center on a regular (every 6 months) basis. Intermittent evaluations should be performed during follow-up visits. This procedure allows for an ongoing evaluation of the patient's progress, as well as of the overall success of the program.

Patient Concerns

It is important that the patient play an active role in developing his or her exercise program, not only with regard to specific exercise preferences, but in understanding and evaluating the effects of exercise on the diabetes and adaptive processes taking place. The patient should be encouraged to check blood glucose regularly and to keep accurate records of glycemic control, diet, exercise, and hypoglycemic occurrences, especially in the initial stages of the exercise program. Hypoglycemia may occur immediately, or maybe 24-48 hours after exercise. Patient glucose monitoring and accurate records help in developing the best insulin, diet, and exercise regimen for the patient.

In order to familiarize the patient with such proper exercise techniques as stretching and heart rate and blood glucose monitoring, it is suggested that all patients go through several initial exercise sessions under supervised conditions (i.e., at the Diabetes Management Center).

Appendix A gives an initial evaluation of Patient X, a sample exercise prescription based on that evaluation, and a sample exercise session that may take place in the Diabetes Management Center.

Clinical Aspects

The private physician should be given a standing order sheet of specific evaluations (the screening procedures previously mentioned) that may be required before the patient begins exercise. Recommendations are given; however, if a fewer or greater number of screening examinations are ordered by the physician, the order should be complied with. The exercise program should be designed with the physician when possible.

Every 3-6 months, the patient should be examined to evaluate adaptation, adherence, and benefits of the exercise program. Glycemic control should be evaluated by glycosylated hemoglobin (HbA_1). When it is possible for the patients to arrive fasted, a lipid profile should be obtained. Height, weight, and insulin dose should be recorded, and the patient should be asked to fill out a simple questionnaire on physical activity patterns, dietary intake, regular blood glucose monitoring, and hypoglycemic occurrences over the past month. Exercise prescriptions should be evaluated and updated at this time.

Risks and Benefits

If a thorough screening examination is performed, and a trained exercise physiologist prescribes an exercise program based on the screening, the risks of regular physical activity are minimal. Risks may include fatigue and muscle soreness during the early stages of exercise; the patient should be instructed on how to stretch and alter the program when necessary. The occurrence of hypoglycemia is a risk for the diabetic participating in exercise; the patient should be counseled on how to avoid hypoglycemia during and after exercise. Benefits of exercise include improved insulin sensitivity, improved glycemic control (Type II's), improved blood lipid profiles, decreased heart rate and blood pressure at rest, decreased body weight, maintenance of lean body mass with weight reduction, and possible decreased risk of premature morbidity and mortality from CHD. It is possible that insulin requirements will be decreased. In addition, improved self-esteem and self-confidence will aid in optimal diabetes management habits of the patient.

Special Precautions

The following are special precautions for exercise prescription for the patient with diabetes:

1. Any patient with retinopathy should avoid strenuous, high-intensity activities that involve breath holding (e.g., weight lifting and isometrics). They should be advised to avoid activities that require lowering the head (e.g., yoga) or that involve jarring of the head.
2. A patient with hypertension should not participate in heavy lifting or breath holding, which increase blood pressure. They should primarily perform dynamic exercises using the large muscle groups (i.e., arms and legs), such as walking and cycling.
3. A patient with insensitive feet (neuropathy) should avoid exercises which traumatize the feet and primarily participate in non-weight-bearing activities, such as swimming and cycling.
4. Every patient should be counseled to examine their feet regularly and treat any abrasions or irritations immediately.
5. Every patient should be advised to be alert for signs of hypoglycemia during and after exercise. Recommendations include:
   - Carry identification with information on diabetes.
   - Carry small carbohydrate source (e.g., candy, dextrose cube, piece of fruit).
   - Exercise when insulin action is not at its peak, preferably after meals or snacks.
   - Monitor blood glucose frequently.
   - Alter insulin dose with guidance of physician; if hypoglycemia is frequent, insulin dose may need reduction.
   - The patient not concerned with weight loss may consume extra carbohydrates prior to and during prolonged exercise, in accordance with the intensity and duration of activity.

6. Every patient should be supplied with information on the caloric requirements of activities to help in choosing proper dietary alterations when indicated. This should be facilitated with nutritional counseling.
7. Other recommendations for the patient include rehydrating carefully (drinking plenty of fluids before, during, and after exercise), and avoiding exercise during the heat of the day and in direct sunlight if possible (wear a hat and sunscreen when indicated).

Appendix A

The following material is an example of an initial patient evaluation. Through such an evaluation, the exercise physiologist can detemine how to familiarize the patient with proper exercise techniques.

Initial Evaluation

Example Case Study: Patient X, a 34-year female, 5'6'', weighing 160 pounds, was seen by private physician on November 1. She was found to have an abnormal oral glucose tolerance test—specifically, fasting blood glucose of 180 mg/dl; at 30 minutes: 300 mg/dl; 60 minutes: 250 mg/dl; 90 minutes: 225 mg/dl; 120 minutes: 200 mg/dl.

This patient had a family history of adult onset diabetes and has experienced an increase in body weight over the past few years. Dr. Y referred Patient X to the Diabetes Management Center for further evaluation and alternative hospitalization according to the multidisciplinary therapeutic care provided by the Center (i.e., dietician, exercise physiologist/specialist, nurse clinician).

Patient X arrived at 8:00 a.m. Monday, November 5, and had a fasting blood sample taken for the determination of glycosylated hemoglobin and blood lipid profile (total cholesterol, triglyceride, low-density lipoprotein cholesterol, and high-density lipoprotein cholesterol). She underwent a cardiovascular exam; a graded exercise test was not indicated (patient less than 35 years of age, no family or personal history of CHD, none of the primary risk factors). Neurological, ophthalmascopic, and nephrological examinations were completed.

The results of the screening evaluation were available by the end of the day. All results were reviewed by the exercise physiologist. HbA$_1$ was elevated: 12.0%. Blood lipid profile revealed elevated triglyceride levels: 250 mg/dl. All other lipid values were normal. Resting heart rate was 70 beats/minutes, and blood pressure was 140/80 mm/hg. No bruits were noted. The ECG was normal. Neurologic, opthalmascopic, and nephrologic examinations were normal. Based on the results and recommendations made by the referring physician, an exercise prescription was developed.

Sample Exercise Prescription

Patient X was given a choice of several aerobic activities to perform (e.g., brisk walking, cycling, aerobics to music). It was agreed upon that brisk walking would be most practical and enjoyable. No musculoskeletal problems were reported that would contraindicate regular brisk walking for Patient X. The program was developed primarily in order to assist in weight loss. Initially this patient will be treated with weight loss and exercise only.

Warm-Up

Light calisthenics (i.e., arm circles and trunk rotations to gradually increase the pulse)

Stimulus

Walking on the treadmill 2.8 mph to attain 136 beats/minute target heart rate (for 5 minutes). Blood pressure was monitored before, during, and after the treadmill exercise session. Patient X was noted to have mildly elevated systolic blood pressure at rest; however, her response to moderate-intensity exercise was normal.

Cool Down

Slowing of walking pace

Stretching and sit-ups

This program would be performed while Patient X is under the care of the center and would be reviewed for continuation at home after she leaves the center. The patient would be instructed to add 2 minutes to the stimulus period each week until she reaches 30 minutes at least three times per week. Blood glucose should be checked by the patient before and after each session to determine the effects of exercise on glycemic control (diet or medications may need alteration when indicated).

References

American College of Sports Medicine. (1986). *Guidelines for graded exercise testing and exercise prescription* (3rd ed.). Philadelphia: Lea and Febiger

American Diabetes Association. (1984). *The physicians guide to Type II diabetes (NIDDM): Diagnosis and treatment*. Alexandria, VA: Author.

Barnard, R.J., Lattimore, L., Holy, R.G., Cherny, S., & Pritikin, N. (1982). Response of non-insulin dependent diabetic patients to an intensive program of diet and exercise. *Diabetes Care, 5*, 370-374.

Blair, S.N., Goodyear, N.N., Gibbons, L.W., & Cooper, K.H. (1984). Physical fitness and incidence of hypertension in healthy normotensive men and women. *Journal of the American Medical Association, 252*, 487-490.

Bogardus, C., Ravussin, L.F., Robbins, D.C., Wolfe, R.R., Horton, E.S., & Sims, E.A.H. (1984). Effects of physical training and diet therapy on carbohydrate metabolism in patients with glucose intolerance and non-insulin dependent diabetes mellitus. *Diabetes, 33*, 311-318.

Campaigne, B.N., Landt, K.W., Mellies, M.J., James, F.W., Glueck, C.J., & Sperling, M.A. (1985). The effects of physical training on blood lipid profiles in adolescents with insulin dependent diabetes mellitus. *The Physician and Sportsmedicine, 13*, 83-89.

Ganda, O.P. (1980). Pathogenesis of macrovascular disease in the human diabetic. *Diabetes, 29*, 931-942.

Goldberg, R.B. (1981). Lipid disorders in diabetes. *Diabetes Care, 4*, 561-572.

Hietanen, E. (Ed.). (1982). *Regulation of serum lipids by physical exercise*. Boca Raton, FL: CRC Press.

LaPorte, R.E., Dorman, J.S., Tajima, N., Cruickshanks, K.J., Orchard, T.J., Cavender, D.E., Becker, D.J., & Drash, A.L. (1986). Pittsburgh insulin-dependent diabetes mellitus morbidity and mortality study: Physical activity and diabetic complications. *Pediatrics, 78*, 1027-1033.

Larsson, Y., Persson, B., Sterky, G., & Thoren, C. (1964). Effects of exercise on blood lipids in juvenile diabetics. *Lancet, 1*, 350-355.

Lingarde, F., & Saltin, B. (1981). Daily physical activity, work capacity, and glucose tolerance in middle-aged men. *Diabetologia, 20*, 134-138.

Miller, N.E., Nesterl, P.J., & Clifton-Bligh, P. (1976). Relationship between plasma lipoprotein cholesterol concentrations and the pool size and metabolism of cholesterol in man. *Atherosclerosis, 23*, 535-547.

Nowalk, N.P., Wing, R.R., Epstein, L.H., Paternostro, M., & Kriska, A. (1983). Exercise intensity in weight loss programs for Type II diabetics. *Diabetes, 33*(Suppl. 1), 19.

Paffenbarger, R.S., Hyde, T.R., Wing, A.L., & Steinmetz, C.H. (1984). A natural history of athleticism and cardiovascular health. *Journal of the American Medical Association, 252*, 491-495.

Pedersen, O., Beck-Neilsen, H., & Heding, L. (1980). Increased insulin receptors after exercise in patients with insulin dependent diabetes mellitus. *New England Journal of Medicine, 302,* 886-892.

Ruderman, N.B., Ganda, O.P., & Johansen, K. (1978). The effect of physical training on glucose tolerance and plasma lipids in maturity onset diabetes. *Diabetes,* **28**(Suppl. 1), 89-92.

Saltin, B., Lindgard, F., Houston, M., Horlin, R., Nygaard, E., & Gad, P. (1979). Physical training and glucose tolerance in middle-aged men with chemical diabetes. *Diabetes,* **28**(Suppl. 1), 30-32.

Schneider, S.H., Amorosa, L.F., Khachadurian, A.K., & Ruderman, N.B. (1984). Studies on the mechanism of improved glucose control during regular exercise in Type II (non-insulin dependent) diabetes. *Diabetologia,* **26,** 355-360.

Trovati, M., Carta, O., Cavalot, F., Vitali, S., Banaudi, C., Lucchina, P.G., Fiocchi, F., Emanuelli, G., & Lenti, G. (1984). Influence of physical training on blood glucose control, glucose tolerance, insulin secretion, and insulin action in non-insulin dependent diabetic patients. *Diabetes Care,* **7,** 416-420.

Wallberg-Henriksson, H., Gunnarsson, R., & Henriksson, J. (1982). Increased peripheral insulin sensitivity and muscle mitochondrial enzymes but unchanged glycemic control in Type I diabetics after physical training. *Diabetes,* **31,** 1044-1050.

Wallberg-Henriksson, H., Gunnarsson, R., Henriksson, J., Ostman, J., & Wahren, J. (1984). Influence of physical training on formation of muscle capillaries in Type I diabetes. *Diabetes,* **33,** 851-857.

Yki-Jarvinen, H., DeFronzo, R., & Koivisto, V.A. (1984). Normalization of insulin sensitivity in Type I diabetic subjects by physical training during insulin pump therapy. *Diabetes Care,* **7,** 520-527.

Zinman, B., Zuniga-Guajardo, S., & Kelly, D. (1984). Comparison of the acute and long-term effects of exercise on glucose control in Type I diabetes. *Diabetes Care,* **7,** 515-519.

The author would like to acknowledge Evelyn Orso and Marti Araujo for the typing of this manuscript.

Chapter 9

Interrelationships of Exercise, Diet, and Medications in Type I and II Diabetes

Marge Samsoe

The triad of factors controlling diabetes includes diet, exercise, and insulin. The insulin may either be the diabetic's own endogenous insulin or injected exogenous insulin. The Type II patient may be using oral hypoglycemic medications in order to enhance cellular insulin sensitivity. Of the three aspects involved with control, only diet instructions are given to all diabetic patients. Prior to the availability of medications, diet and exercise were the only means of attempting to control diabetes. Exercise has become more popular for the entire population over the last decade. It is the portion of the patient's treatment regimen which is the most "normal" to do. For patients in whom diabetic control cannot be achieved with a combination of diet and exercise, medications are added.

The primary emphasis in this presentation is on increasing a person's exercise in a systematic manner, for this is a topic that is inadequately covered in most other resources. The areas to be covered include the benefits of exercise, contraindications to exercise, types of exercise, timing of exercise, precautions with exercise, adjustments in diabetes treatment resulting from change in exercise, and how to progress with exercise for the patient.

Benefits of Exercise

There are many benefits of exercise, both generally and specifically for diabetics. Primarily, the chosen type of exercise needs to be enjoyable; otherwise, participation will not be continued on a regular basis. Physical activity can be an opportunity to share an invigorating experience with friends. Exercise firms the muscles being used, therefore improving body tone and possibly decreasing body size. A loss of inches with exercise is usually seen prior to actual weight loss. Because of the increased caloric expenditure, weight loss may occur if caloric intake is not increased to compensate. As the metabolic rate is increased, a person's energy level may also increase. The change of pace from routine daily work activities may also provide a psychological release. These advantages of exercise are applicable to all active people, regardless of whether they have diabetes. Health care professionals prescribing exercise for patients should also engage in regular exercise so they can be believable to their patients.

Because of the twofold increase in cardiac disease among diabetics, the cardiovascular benefits of exercise are even more important for them than for the general population. These benefits have been thoroughly discussed and debated in the literature. Exercise may or may not increase longevity; however, it probably increases quality of life. These are the primary cardiovascular benefits:

- Decreased resting heart rate and blood pressure
- Decreased heart rate and systolic blood pressure with submaximal work
- Increased myocardial blood flow reserve
- Faster return to resting heart rate after exercise
- Increased high density lipoproteins (HDL)
- Decreased cholesterol
- Decreased triglycerides

A specific benefit of exercise for the diabetic is that it enhances glucose utilization, due to an increase in insulin sensitivity. Muscle glucose uptake is enhanced as long as the individual is already adequately insulinized (Soman, Koivisto, Deibert, Felig, & De Fronzo, 1979). The mechanism of this appears to be that the capillary surface area is increased. Insulin sensitivity is enhanced, although the mechanism here is unclear. In order for exercise to have an advantageous effect on blood glucose, one must begin with a level below 250 mg/dl, for reasons that will be discussed later. Exercise also increases insulin binding to receptors (Roth, 1981).

Exercise allows the body to make better use of available insulin (Pederson, Beck-Nielsen, & Heding, 1980). This can be the patient's own insulin or that which is injected. If the person is non-insulin-dependent (Type II), exercise may spare the beta cells of the pancreas and allow the patient to control the diabetes with diet and exercise alone, rather than having to resort to using oral hypoglycemic agents or exogenous insulin. If the person is using diabetic medications, the amount required may be reduced (Costill, Miller, & Fink, 1980). When exercise is added to diet to help control diabetes, glucose disposal increases significantly (Figure 1; Bogardus et al., 1984). In the well-insulinized diabetic, even prolonged exercise (up

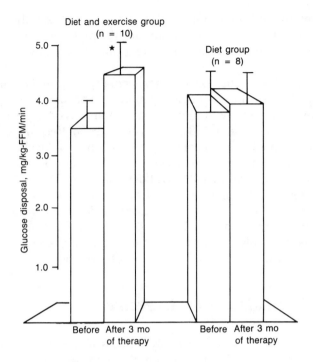

Figure 1 The euglycemic clamp is a measurement of the body's sensitivity to infused insulin. Insulin is infused to maintain a constant (high) plasma insulin level, and a variable amount of glucose is infused to keep the plasma glucose level constant. The amount of glucose infused is an index of tissue sensitivity to insulin. Total glucose disposal, or "M" value (as determined by the euglycemic clamp) before and after 3 months of treatment with diet alone or diet plus exercise. *Note*. From "Diet and Exercise: Important Therapeutic Tools" by T.J. Devlin and E.S. Horton, 1984, *Drug Therapy*, p. 114. Adapted from "Effects of Physical Training and Diet Therapy on Carbohydrate Metabolism in Patients With Glucose Intolerance and Non-Insulin Dependent Diabetes Mellitus" by C. Bogardus et al., 1984, *Diabetes*, **33**. Reproduced with permission from the American Diabetes Association, Inc.

FFM = fat free mass.

*Significant increase in total glucose disposal in this group, $p < 0.05$.

to 4 hours) can be accomplished under metabolic conditions similar to those of non-diabetics.

Exercise is not the primary therapy for Type I (insulin-dependent) diabetics. Their metabolic control must be achieved mainly by balancing exogenous insulin with food intake. In fact, exercise, particularly if done on an irregular basis, may compound problems with blood glucose control. However, these patients do benefit from all of the social and cardiovascular advantages of exercise. Many of them desire to exercise, and they must understand the metabolic effects of their chosen exercise in order to be successful and comfortable. Diabetics have successfully completed marathon runs (26.2 miles) and triathlons (2.4 mile swim plus 112 mile bicycle ride plus 26.2 mile run). Planning prior to such events needs to be meticulous.

For the Type II diabetic, exercise may actually be more beneficial than for the Type I. The primary problem generally is being overweight. Exercise can be used along with diet to facilitate improved control with the compliant patient (Beeken, 1980; Saltin et al., 1979). Recent studies have shown that fasting blood glucose and hemoglobin A_{1c} levels decrease in Type II diabetics following exercise training programs ranging from 3-8 months (Devlin & Horton, 1984; Krotkiewski, 1984). Trovati's group recently showed improvement in blood glucose control, as evidenced by improved hemoglobin A_{1c}, fasting plasma glucose, and fasting plasma insulin in diet-controlled Type II diabetics (Trovati, et al., 1984). Cardiovascular disease is also very prevalent in this group; exercise may help to decrease the risk of serious cardiovascular disease.

Contraindications to Exercise

Generally speaking, exercise actually reduces blood glucose in the diabetic (Wahren, 1979). The decrease in blood glucose following injected insulin and rest, in comparison with injected insulin and exercise, can be seen in Figure 2 (Lawrence, 1926). In contrast to this, if blood glucose exceeds 250-300 mg/dl prior to exercise, and insulin is not injected, the blood glucose may actually rise. This usually occurs in the Type I diabetic who has an inadequate amount of insulin available. Since there is an insufficient amount of insulin present, the normal process of accelerated glucose uptake and utilization by the muscle is inhibited. Hepatic glucose production is then unrestrained, resulting in an increased rise in blood glucose with exercise. This may also be exaggerated due to increases in counterregulatory hormones (especially catecholamines and growth hormones) (Brownless & Flassor, 1982). A summary of the effects of exercise on nondiabetics in comparison with diabetics, regarding various parameters in the blood, muscle, and liver, can be seen in Table 1 (Ludvigsson, 1980). The effects of exercise on blood glucose and plasma ketones are graphically presented in Figure 3 (Devlin & Horton, 1984). The effects of exercise on catecholamines and growth hormones are delineated in Figure 4 (Koivisto & Felig, 1981; Tamborlane, 1979).

The patient should also not begin exercise while hypoglycemic. Blood glucose needs to be at least 80 mg/dl and may need to be somewhat higher, depending on the duration and intensity of the anticipated exercise. With the increase of home blood glucose monitoring, it is much easier for a patient to determine the appropriateness of exercise and its effects.

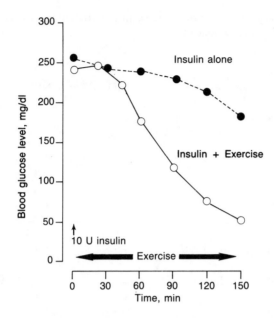

Figure 2 Effect of subcutaneously injected insulin and muscular exercise on blood glucose levels in a juvenile diabetic patient. *Note.* From "The Effects of Exercise on Insulin Action in Diabetes" by R.D. Lawrence, 1926, *British Medical Journal, 1,* p. 648. Copyright 1926 by the British Medical Association. Reprinted by permission.

Also, more patients are changing to multiple injections throughout the day, which allows for more flexibility in planning.

The diabetic must take exemplary care of the feet. If there is a blister, cut, or infection present, weight-bearing exercise is contraindicated. This is because of the increased susceptibility to infection, gangrene, and slow healing, particularly in the diabetic whose blood glucose is frequently elevated. The patient must be taught to examine the feet before and after exercise. Frequently, sensation in the extremities is decreased due to peripheral neuropathy, making the foot checks all the more important. Prior to exercise, the inside of shoes also need to be examined for any foreign objects which might have fallen into them and might cause harm to insensitive feet. With the diabetic patient, progression from injury to infection to gangrene to amputation can take place quite rapidly—as fast as 7-10 days. The patient must be particularly aware of this fact. If there is significant neuropathy, it also might be difficult to complete an adequate amount of weight-bearing exercise. For this person it might be more appropriate to use bicycling or swimming as the primary exercise.

If the patient has diabetic retinopathy, further precautions must be taken in order not to exacerbate this condition. Primarily, one is trying to prevent abrupt or pronounced elevations in the blood pressure, because this

Table 1   Summary of Effects of Exercise in Nondiabetics, Nonketotic Diabetics, and Ketotic Diabetics

Systemic Factor Affected by Exercise	ND[a]	NKD[b]	KD[c]
Blood			
Glucose	(−)	−	+ +
FFA	+	+ +	+ + +
Ketones	+	+ +	+ + +
Muscle			
Glucose uptake	+	+	+
FFA uptake	+	+	+ + +
Ketone uptake	0	+	+ + +
Postexercise glycogen synthesis	+ + +	+ + +	+
Liver			
Glucose output	+	+	+
Glycogenolysis	+	+ +	+ +
Gluconeogenesis	(+)	+ +	+ + +
Ketone production	0	+	+ + +

Note. From "Scandinavian Symposium: Physical Exercise in the Treatment of Juvenile Diabetes Mellitus" by J. Ludvigsson (Ed.), 1980, *Acta Paediatrica Scandinavica*, **69**(Suppl. 283), p. 121. Copyright 1980 by Almqvist and Wiksell Int. Adapted by permission.

− = decrease; +, + +, + + + = varying degrees of increment; 0 = nonexistent.
[a]ND = nondiabetics. [b]NKD = nonketotic diabetics. [c]KD = ketotic diabetics.

can actually cause a retinal hemorrhage. The type of retinopathy must be determined by the patient's ophthalmologist.

The patient with nonproliferative retinopathy may do all non-Valsalva exercises, including swimming, jogging, bicycling, and racquet sports. Those activities which are contraindicated generally invoke the Valsalva reflex or abruptly increase the blood pressure and include bowling (Valsalva), yoga (particularly those positions bearing weight on the head), weight lifting, and advanced Nautilus.

When a patient has proliferative retinopathy, activities must be further restricted in order not to exacerbate the condition. Otherwise, blindness can result! If blood pressure control is excellent, the individual may swim (with good breathing technique, rather than holding the breath), jog lightly, or bicycle easily. Contraindicated are diving, bowling, yoga, Nautilus, push-ups, sit-ups, activities with the head below the waist, strenuous jogging or bicycling, racquet sports, and advanced isometrics. The patient with neovascularization can usually tolerate a systolic blood

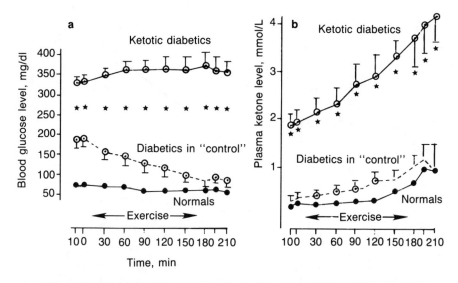

Figure 3 Effect of prolonged exercise on (a) blood glucose levels and (b) plasma ketone bodies (acetoacetate and 3-hydroxybutyrate) in healthy control subjects, diabetic patients in moderate metabolic control, and in ketotic diabetic patients. Circled values in the diabetic patients are significantly different from corresponding values of the control group (p < .05). Stars indicate statistically significant differences (p < .05) between corresponding values of the two groups of diabetic patients. *Note*. From "Diet and Exercise: Important Therapeutic Tools" by J.T. Devlin and E.S. Horton, 1984, *Drug Therapy*, **14**, p. 113. Adapted from "Metabolic and Hormonal Effects of Muscular Exercise in Juvenile Type Diabetes" by G.M. Berchtold et al., 1977, *Diabetologia*, **13**, p. 355.

pressure of 140-160. Following laser photocoagulation, the patient should continue using the same guidelines as for proliferative retinopathy.

Types of Exercise

Aerobic exercise is the best type of exercise for achieving cardiovascular benefits. It is also the best for smoothing out daily overall blood glucose levels. Aerobic exercises include such activities as walking, running, bicycling, swimming, and cross-country skiing. In order to be of cardiovascular benefit, the exercise must be sustained at an intensity which will keep the heart rate elevated to a prescribed level (approximately 60-85% of the heart rate reserve, if it is known) for a minimum of 20-30 minutes at least three times per week. This is the minimum level, better results can be seen when the amount of time per session and the frequency per week is increased.

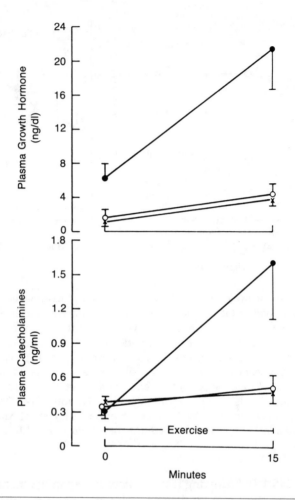

Figure 4 Plasma growth hormone and catecholamine (epinephrine plus norepinephrine) response to 15-minute exercise in healthy controls (x) and in insulin-dependent diabetics during conventional treatment (φ) and in the same patients after 2 weeks of treatment (o) with a portable, subcutaneous insulin infusion system. *Note.* From ''Exercise in Diabetes: Clinic Implications'' by V.A. Koivisto and P. Felig, 1981, in H. Rifkin and P. Raskin (Eds.), *Diabetes Mellitus, Vol. V* (p. 142), Bowie, MD: Brady. Reproduced with permission from the American Diabetes Association, Inc.

For the diabetic patient, better control can be achieved by doing a similar amount of exercise at approximately the same time each day. This is particularly true for the diabetic using insulin, because the amount of insulin needed throughout the day and the meal plan may need readjusting with a change in exercise. The patient may have variety in the types of activities done, but it is helpful if the overall caloric expenditure is similar. For this reason the "Exercise Exchange System" was developed (Table 2).

Other activities with caloric expenditure calculated may also be incorporated for a patient. Many people wish to do other activities which are not aerobic in nature, such as tennis, softball, and golf. These activities are somewhat less predictable in their energy expenditure and do not have the cardiovascular advantages of aerobics. Nonetheless, they are just as important for the social aspects and still increase caloric expenditure. Table 3 indicates caloric expenditure for various activities.

For patients doing acute, intense exercise, such as sprinting, blood glucose may increase. This is caused by the increase in catecholamines with this type of exercise. The patient needs to be aware of this so as not to get discouraged.

Many people have difficulty fitting exercise into an already crowded daily schedule. Often exercise can be incorporated into normal daily activities. It might be feasible to walk or ride a bicycle to work; if the distance is too great, there is still no law requiring employees to use the parking spot closest to the building where they are going. If a person parks a mile away, there is probably less parking hassle, and automatically he or she has walked an extra 2 miles a day! Many times, using the stairs is faster than waiting for an elevator, and climbing the stairs gradually becomes easier.

It is not always practical for a person to exercise daily at the same time and for the same duration. In this case, the person needs to learn approximately how much a given amount of exercise affects his or her blood glucose level and how to readjust the insulin dose or meal covering that time period. It is important to realize, though, that all diabetic patients do not respond the same to a given amount of exercise and that individuals may respond differently on different days. There are many things

Table 2 Exercise Exchange System

Activity	Distance or Duration
Walking	1 mile
Jogging	1 mile
Bicycling	3 miles
Skiing cross-country	3/4 mile
Swimming	About 10-14 minutes (depends on swimming skill)

Note. Each activity uses about 100 calories for a 150-pound person.

Table 3 Calories Burned in Various Physical Activities

Work Activities	Calories per Minute	Recreational Activities	Calories per Minute
Clerical work	1.2-1.6	Cycling (5-15 mph, 10-speed bicycle	5.0-12.0
Farming			
Chores	3.8	Running	
Planting, hoeing, raking	4.7	12-min mile (5 mph)	10.0
Gardening		8-min mile	15.0
Digging	8.6	(7.5 mph)	
Weeding	5.6	6-min mile	20.0
Hiking		(10 mph)	
Road-field (3.5 mph)	5.6-7.0	Skiing	
Uphill: 5-15% grade (3.5 mph)	8.0-15.0	Moderate to steep (downhill)	8.0-12.0
House painting	3.5	Cross-country (3-8 mph)	9.0-17.0
Sawing		Swimming	
Chain saw	6.2	Pleasure	6.0
		Crawl (25-50 yd/ min)	6.0-12.5
		Skipping rope	10.0-15.0

affecting a person's blood glucose in addition to exercise, diet, and medication, such as stress in various forms and subclinical illness.

In establishing an exercise program for a patient who previously has been inactive, one must begin slowly and progress steadily, particularly with someone over the age of 30. This decreases the likelihood of the patient developing an overuse injury and gives the person confidence in increasing ability. The programs developed for cardiac rehabilitation have excellent guidelines. A basic walking program should begin at whatever distance the person is currently walking and increase about 2/10 mile per day to 1 mile. After a week at this level, another increase can be made at 2/10 mile per day to 2 miles. This level also should be maintained for at least one week before again increasing 2/10 mile per day to 3 miles, which is a good target distance. Before the person begins to run, if that is the goal, he or she should be able to walk 3 miles without difficulty; this will decrease the likelihood of musculoskeletal injuries. Other activities may be increased using a similar program.

When one is doing stationary bicycling, an adequate goal is 30 minutes of continuous riding, divided so that the first 5 minutes is at a very light resistance for warm-up; followed by 20 minutes at a level of resistance intense enough to achieve the target heart rate; the final 5 minutes should be a cool-down with very light resistance, in order to return the heart rate and blood pressure gradually to pre-exercise levels. As the level of conditioning improves, more resistance can be applied during the resistance portion, but the length of time really does not need to be increased.

Timing of Exercise

In order for exercise to be of greatest value and to cause the least discomfort, the time of day during which the exercise session takes place is an important consideration. If exercise is done about 1-1 1/2 hours following a meal, it can decrease the postprandial rise in blood glucose (Caron, Poussier, Marliss, & Zinman, 1982). This is beneficial for both types of diabetes. Exercise at this time is unlikely to cause an insulin reaction in patients using insulin. If a patient is on a split dose of insulin, using regular and NPH insulin, the peaks of insulin action and blood glucose would be as shown in Figure 5. Ideally the exercise should be inserted into the

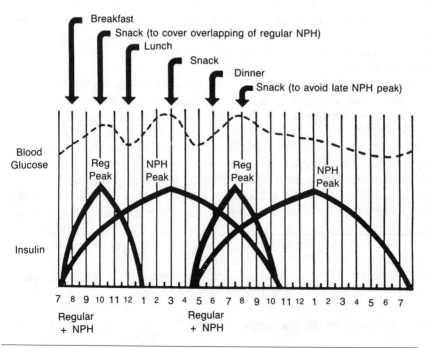

Figure 5 Blood glucose and insulin peaks, showing how insulin can help cover meal and snack pattern.

daily schedule before or at the peaks. If the exercise takes place follow-ing a peak, the individual using the insulin will need to make some management changes in order to avoid an insulin reaction.

It is always necessary for the person to have a rapid-acting carbohydrate available in case of an insulin reaction. Some items easy to carry are 6-ounce cans of juice, small packages of raisins (2 tablespoons fit in a canister from 35 mm film), six packets of sugar (in a plastic bag to loop over a waistband), one small tube of cake gel, and any of the commercial items to raise blood sugar, such as Glucose Tablets, Glutose, Instant Glu-cose, and Monojel. One word of caution: If exercise is going to be in very cold conditions, be sure the item chosen does not freeze!

Depending on the time and amount of exercise, it might also be ap-propriate to have a supplemental snack 20-30 minutes prior to exercise. This is particularly important for the person who is exercising prior to a meal. It is common to desire to exercise after work or school and before the evening meal. This is the usual time for athletic practice for school athletic teams. With exercise at this time, the patient must make adjust-ments in overall management in order to avoid hypoglycemia.

Blood glucose can continue to decrease for up to 5 hours following ex-ercise. Every patient needs to be well aware of this. It can result in an insulin reaction right before the next meal. This meal may be several hours after the exercise, making it difficult for the patient to relate the reaction to the exercise session, unless there is prior knowledge of this effect. In addition, the blood glucose may remain lowered for 24-48 hours (Zinman, Vranic, Albisser, Leibel, & Marliss, 1979). This helps out overall control, but may cause difficulties initially in rearranging the patient's total treat-ment program.

Depending on the type of exercise, the area of insulin injection may be important. Insulin injected over a muscle that is being used for the activity may be more rapidly absorbed (Richter, Ruderman, & Schneider, 1981; Skyler, 1979). If a patient is going to be walking, running, or bi-cycling, it would not be advisable to use the thigh for an injection site prior to activity. Figure 6 demonstrates glycemic response to using the thigh and arm as injection sites during leg exercise, in contrast to no ex-ercise (Zinman et al., 1977). Likewise, if the person is going to be playing tennis or canoeing, the tricep area is inappropriate. Following exercise there is increased glucose uptake in the muscles that were used. It is not currently known what effect this has on the choice of an injection site following exercise. Generally speaking, the abdomen is a safe injection site. Absorption from abdominal injections is more rapid than other areas, but is less likely to be affected by exercise.

Precautions With Exercise

For diabetics using insulin, the symptoms for an insulin reaction may be different with exercise from those experienced while less active. The usual

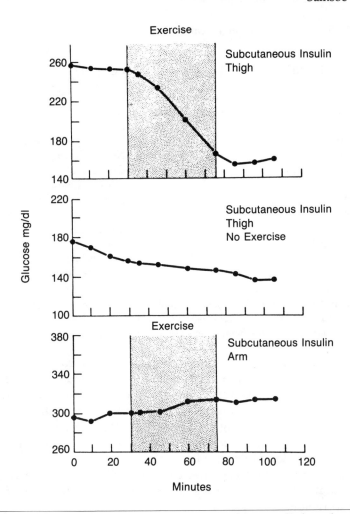

Figure 6 Glycemic response to exercise in one subject studied on three separate occasions. 1) Insulin injected subcutaneously (sc) in an exercising thigh (upper panel). 2) Insulin sc in the thigh without exercise (middle panel). 3) Insulin into an immobilized arm during exercise (lower panel). *Note.* From B. Zinman et al., "Glucoregulation During Moderate Exercise in Insulin-Treated Diabetics," *Journal of Clinical Endocrinology and Metabolism,* Volume 45, p. 648, © by the Endocrine Society, 1977.

initial symptoms may be masked. The general symptoms for hypoglycemia are outlined in Table 4.

Sweating, increased heart rate, and fatigue are expected with exercise. Hunger and hand tremors are usually not perceived during strenuous exercise. Irritability is often perceived better by those around the person than by himself. By the time the individual is dizzy, feeling faint, confused, or uncoordinated, intervention with a fast-acting carbohydrate is

Table 4   Symptoms of Hypoglycemia

Catecholamine Release Related	Cerebral Glucose Deprivation
Sweating	Apathy
Excessive hunger	Headache
Hand tremors	Inability to concentrate
Palpitations	Nervousness
Drowsiness, fatigue	Circumoral paresthesias
Dizziness	Blurred vision
Irritability	Poor coordination
Faintness	Personality changes
Crying	Slurred speech
Unsteady gait	Convulsions
	Confusion
	Unconsciousness

Note. From "Hypoglycemia in Diabetic Patients and Clinical Recognition of Those at Risk" by F.W. Whitehouse, 1983, *Practical Cardiology,* **9**, p. 196, 199. Copyright 1983. Adapted from *Practical Cardiology* with permission.

needed quickly to prevent a further drop in blood glucose, which could result in unconsciousness. (An unconscious person should never be given liquids or food.) With, or following, exercise, it is also possible for the symptoms to progress more rapidly than usual, because the blood glucose level may be dropping quickly. Uncomfortable and pronounced symptoms can be prevented or alleviated by careful monitoring and prompt intervention when needed.

A patient using beta-blocker medications may have blunted perception of the initial symptoms of an insulin reaction. The patient needs to be careful to monitor blood glucose.

Dehydration may be more of a problem for diabetics than the general population, especially with activities of long duration in the heat or at high altitude. This is of particular concern for the diabetic who is hyperglycemic and may actually be dehydrated prior to exercise. This can be alleviated by having good glycemic control prior to exercise and by taking plenty of fluids during the activity.

The most important equipment for any activity in which there is weight bearing are the shoes. They must fit well and be properly padded, in order to prevent blisters and provide support. Running shoes are the best shoes for either walking or running. If the activity involves lateral movements, such as in tennis or basketball, then shoes designed for those sports are necessary. When a person gets new shoes, they should be broken in gradually.

Every person with diabetes should wear a diabetic identification bracelet or neck chain. This is very important should the person become unconscious as a result of hypoglycemia, hyperglycemia, or an accident. This type of identification facilitates treatment more rapidly than identification in a wallet, which may not be found.

It is a good idea to exercise with another person. This adds to one's enjoyment and provides an element of safety in the event of an accident or an insulin reaction. Obviously, the friend needs to be informed of the diabetic's usual symptoms for an insulin reaction and what actions should be taken if the diabetic does experience hypoglycemia. However, it is best to be totally responsible for one's own diabetic control. Good control gives an increased feeling of self-confidence and freedom. If an individual depends on others to watch for symptoms, it may lead to irresponsibility.

Adjustments in Treatments

Diabetic control is achieved through a balance of diet, exercise, and sometimes medication (insulin or oral hypoglycemic agents). If one aspect, e.g., exercise, is changed, the other two areas must also be modified if a steady state is desired. There are two options in this case: Either the total calories of the diet can be increased or the medication can be decreased (Peterson et al., 1979). The determination of which is appropriate must be based on the individual patient. If the person is thin, it would be desirable to increase the food intake with exercise and continue the same medications. On the contrary, if the person is overweight and using insulin or oral agents, usually it would be most appropriate to reduce these and maintain the same diet (Vramic & Berger, 1979). If the medications are maintained steady in the patient, weight loss will not be accomplished with exercise, due to the necessity of increasing food intake in order to prevent hypoglycemia. For the overweight, diet-controlled diabetic, it would be best to make no other modification and to expect a negative caloric balance.

Obviously, if changes are going be required in the eating or medication pattern or both, it would be most desirable for the person to exercise on a regular basis, so everything doesn't have to be juggled every day. This is to be encouraged, but is not always practical. When there is an irregular schedule, the diabetic must adhere closely to careful testing in order to make educated decisions on management changes. Some patients can develop two basic programs, one for active days and one for sedentary days.

Some diabetics are attempting such long-distance aerobic activities as running marathons (26.2 miles), bicycle touring (50-100 miles per day), and cross country ski touring (10-50 miles). If proper precautions and training are made, these endurance activities are possible and can be enjoyable. There is currently little research in this area. Most of the time it is an experiment of one, in that each person responds uniquely. The individual must closely monitor the blood glucose responses to various

Table 5   Exercise to Exhaustion

Times	Group	A	B	C	D
7:30 a.m.	Insulin (% of usual dose)	100	100	50	20
8:00 a.m.	Food (% of usual intake)	100	100	100	100
9:00 a.m.	Exercise time to exhaustion	60'	70'	80'	180'

Note. From "Exercise and Diabetes Mellitus: Physical Activity as a Part of Daily Life and Its Role in the Treatment of Diabetic Patients" by F.W. Kemmer and M. Berger, 1983, *International Journal of Sports Medicine,* **4**, p. 83. Copyright 1983 by George Thieme Verlag. Adapted by permission.

regimens of exercise intensity and duration, as well as the amount of food eaten prior to the event and the food consumed during the event. As previously mentioned, the blood glucose must not exceed 250 mg/dl prior to beginning the exercise. Because of the number of calories used during the activity, care must be taken to have adequate blood glucose prior to starting. In a study by Kemmer and Berger (1983), it was found that endurance exercise could be continued for the longest period of time if the athlete decreased his or her insulin to only 20% of the usual dose prior to the event. The results of this study are seen in Table 5.

With prolonged exercise, symptomatic hypoglycemia is more likely to occur. First, the blood glucose concentration decreases (Skyler, 1979). Next, the hepatic glycogen stores are depleted. The next available route for fuel is through hepatic gluconeogenesis, which is a slower method of generating glucose (Ruderman, Young, & Schneider, 1984). The distance athlete needs to be aware of this.

It is possible for the diabetic using insulin to carbohydrate load, if desired, by increasing the insulin slightly the day before the event, along with increasing carbohydrate consumption the day of the event. Again, care must be taken to monitor blood glucose. During the exercise, carbohydrates generally may be consumed as tolerated without significant elevations in blood glucose.

If a patient is hospitalized to attain or regain diabetic control, the person's activities should be as similar as possible to those at home. This may even be a good time to show the person the values of exercise through walking and bicycling. However if a person is inactive in the hospital and is using any diabetic medications, problems of hypoglycemia may occur upon returning to a more active lifestyle at home (Jette, 1984).

The improvements from exercise that are seen in glucose homeostasis are rapidly lost within a 2-week period if exercise is stopped. Therefore, it is important for the person to maintain regular exercise. It has been shown that high-school- and college-age diabetics have a lower exercise tolerance than the general population (Larsson, 1980). This is probably due to overprotection, lack of exercise, and fear of insulin reactions, rather than to the actual effects of diabetes in these age groups. Most of these persons are capable of attaining above-normal fitness levels if they follow a sound exercise program. There are, however, some physiological parameters that can actually result in a decreased ability to exchange oxygen at the cellular level. Erythrocytes do not deform as readily in diabetics, making oxygen exchange more difficult in the capillary and venous systems. Also, gas diffusion is less efficient when the basement membrane is thicker, as is common in diabetics (McMillan, 1979). With regular exercise and careful glucose monitoring, the basement membrane decreases in thickness (Peterson, Jones, Esterly, Wantz, & Jackson, 1980).

Protocol for Exercise Prescription for Diabetics

The following was developed for use with patients at Gundersen Clinic, Ltd., in La Crosse, Wisconsin. It would need to be modified for other groups to use, depending on the specific situations.

The initial evaluation and referral for exercise should be done by the person's physician. The person's overall glycemic control should be assessed. The home blood glucose (or urine) testing records should be reviewed. A glycosylated hemoglobin may be done to assess overall control. The patient should be carefully examined for such complications of diabetes as cardiovascular problems, neuropathy, retinopathy, and nephropathy. The patient's current exercise tolerance should be determined. This can best be done with a graded exercise test using either a treadmill or bicycle ergometer along with electrocardiographic and blood pressure monitoring. This is important, in order to determine the possibility of latent cardiovascular disease and to make an appropriate exercise prescription (Leon et al., 1984). If the patient is planning to use a stationary bicycle at home, testing should be done on the bicycle ergometer for the patient with diabetic retinopathy, as blood pressure response with cycling is usually higher than with walking.

The exercise prescription must take into consideration the types of activities which the person enjoys, along with any limitations which he or she might have. The prescription basics are set up with attention to frequency, intensity, and duration of the exercise, along with special consideration for the time of day of the exercise. The person's goals for exercise, weight, and diabetic control must be thoroughly determined, assessed, and put into reasonable perspective. Modifications in diet or medications, along with precautions to be taken, must be discussed.

The person should be aware of the tangible results of exercise that can be experienced, such as short-term decrease in blood glucose, long-term improvement in blood glucose control, increased exercise tolerance, improvement in blood lipids, and lowered blood pressure. These parameters should be measured at appropriate intervals to see how well the patient is accomplishing the goals set. Reevaluation frequency needs to be individually determined.

Some patients require more elaborate testing and monitoring to establish safe and effective programs. On several occasions we have done blood glucose determinations before and after exercise, and again 3-5 hours later, in order to determine what effect the exercise has on a patient's blood glucose level. This has allowed for better fine-tuning of the change in insulin dose (primarily for the Type I diabetic).

It also should be mentioned that all patients do not always respond to exercise in the expected manner, nor is the response always reliably reproducible. This can be very frustrating. The diabetic needs to know that there can be fluctuations in blood glucose caused by stress or low-grade infection, besides by mismanagement. Stress can be very hard to predict or manage.

Summary

Exercise can be helpful in the overall management of the patient with diabetes, particularly Type II. It can help to lower and smooth out blood glucose levels. In addition, it can build confidence in the person who has accomplished goals that have been set. For the Type I diabetic, exercise is certainly possible and desirable, as long as the patient learns the necessary management techniques. There are several precautions that should be taken in order to make exercise a safe and enjoyable experience. Exercise should be an enjoyable portion of the diabetic's life. For nearly every patient, the effects of exercise are desirable and attainable.

References

Beeken, R.K. (1980). Initiating exercise programs for patients with non-insulin-dependent diabetes. *Diabetes Care*, **3**, 627-628.

Bogardus, C., Ravussin, E., Robbins, D., Wolfe, R., Horton, E., & Sims, E. (1984). Effects of physical training and diet therapy on carbohydrate metabolism in patients with glucose intolerance and non-insulin-dependent diabetes mellitus. *Diabetes*, **33**, 311-318.

Brownlee, M., & Flassor, H. (1982). Exercise and the diabetic patient. *Drug Therapy*, **12**(3), 66-72.

Caron, D., Poussier, P., Marliss, E., & Zinman, B. (1982). The effect of postprandial exercise on meal-related glucose intolerance in insulin-dependent diabetic individuals. *Diabetes Care*, **5**, 364-374.

Costill, D.L., Miller, J.M., & Fink, W.J. (1980). Energy metabolism in diabetic distance runners. *The Physician and Sports Medicine*, **8**(10), 63-71.

Devlin, J.T., & Horton, E.S. (1984). Diet and exercise: Important theraeutic tools. *Drug Therapy*, **14**(3), 109-115.

Jette, D.U. (1984). Physical effects of exercise in the diabetic. *Physical Therapy*, **64**, 339-342.

Kemmer, F.W., & Berger, M. (1983). Exercise and diabetes mellitus: Physical activity as a part of daily life and its role in the treatment of diabetic patients. *International Journal of Sports Medicine*, **4**, 77-88.

Koivisto, V.A., & Felig, P. (1981). Exercise in diabetes: Clinical complications. In H. Rifkin & P. Raskin (Eds.), *Diabetes mellitus* (Vol. 5; pp. 137-144). Bowie, MD: Brady.

Krotkiewski, M. (1984). Physical training in the prophylaxis and treatment of obesity, hypertension, and diabetes. *Scandinavian Journal of Rehabilitation Medicine*, **9**, 55-70.

Krzentowski, G., Pirnay, F., Pallikarakis, N., Luycka, A., Lacroix, M., Mosora, F., & Lefèbure, P. (1981). Glucose utilization during exercise in normal and diabetic subjects: The role of insulin. *Diabetes*, **30**, 983-989.

Larsson, Y. (1980). Physical exercise and juvenile diabetes: Summary and conclusions. *Acta Paediatrica Scandinavica*, **69**(Suppl. 283), 120-122.

Lawrence, R.D. (1926). The effects of exercise on insulin action in diabetes. *British Medical Journal*, **1**, 648-650.

Leon, A.S., Conrad, J., Casal, D., Serfass, R., Bonnard, R., Goetz, F., & Blackburn, H. (1984). Exercise for diabetics: Effects of conditioning at constant body weight. *Journal of Cardiac Rehabilitation*, **64**, 278-286.

Ludvigsson, J. (Ed.) (1980). Scandinavian symposium: Physical exercise in the treatment of juvenile diabetes mellitus. *Acta Paediatrica Scandinavica*, **69**(Suppl. 283), 1-122.

McMillan, D.E. (1979). Exercise and diabetic microangiopathy. *Diabetes*, **28**(Suppl. 1), 103-105.

Pedersen, O., Beck-Nielsen, H., & Heding, L. (1980). Increased insulin receptors after exercise in patients with insulin-dependent diabetes mellitus. *New England Journal of Medicine*, **302**, 886-891.

Peterson, C.M., Jones, R., Dupuis, A., Levin, B., Bernstein, R., & O'Shea, M. (1979). Feasibility of improved blood glucose control in patients with insulin-dependent diabetes mellitus. *Diabetes Care*, **2**, 329-335.

Peterson, C.M., Jones, R., Esterly, J., Wantz, G., & Jackson, R. (1980). Changes in basement membrane thickening and pulse volume concomitant with improved glucose control and exercise in patients with insulin-dependent diabetes mellitus. *Diabetes Care*, **3**, 586-589.

Richter, E.A., Ruderman, N.B., & Schneider, S.H. (1981). Diabetes and exercise. *American Journal of Medicine*, **70**, 201-209.

Roth, J. (1981). Insulin binding to its receptor: Is the receptor more important than the hormone? *Diabetes Care*, **4**, 27-32.

Ruderman, N.B., Young, J.C., & Schneider, S.H. (1984). Exercise as a therapeutic tool in the Type I diabetic. *Practical Cardiology*, **10**, 143-153.

Saltin, B., Lindgärde, F., Houston, M., Hörlin, R., Nygaard, E., & Gad, P. (1979). Physical training and glucose tolerance in middle-aged men with chemical diabetes. *Diabetes*, **28**(Suppl. 1), 30-42.

Skyler, J.S. (1979). Diabetes and exercise: Clinical implications. *Diabetes Care*, **2**, 307-311.

Soman, V.R., Koivisto, V., Deibert, D., Felig, P., & DeFronzo, R. (1979). Increased insulin sensitivity and insulin binding to monocytes after physical training. *New England Journal of Medicine*, **301**, 1200-1204.

Tamborlane, W.V. (1979). Normalization of growth hormone and catecholamine response to exercise in juvenile onset diabetes treated with a portable insulin infusion pump. *Diabetes*, **28**, 785-788.

Trovati, M., Carta, Q., Cavalot, F., Vitali, S., Banaudi, C., Lucchina, P., Fiocchi, F., Emanuelli, G., & Lenti, G. (1984). Influence of physical training on blood glucose control, glucose tolerance, insulin secretion, and insulin action in non-insulin-dependent diabetic patients. *Diabetes Care*, **7**, 416-420.

Vramic, M., & Berger, M. (1983). Exercise and diabetes mellitus. *Diabetes*, **28**, 147-163.

Wahren, J. (1979). Glucose turnover during exercise in healthy man and in patients with diabetes mellitus. *Diabetes*, **28**(Suppl. 1), 82-88.

Whitehouse, F.W. (1983). Hypoglycemia in diabetic patients and clinical recognition of those at risk. *Practical Cardiology*, **9**, 195-205.

Zinman, B., Murray, F., Vranic, M., Albisser, A., Leibel, B., McClean, P., & Marliss, E. (1977). Glucoregulation during moderate exercise in insulin treated diabetics. *Journal of Clinical Endrocrinology and Metabolism*, **45**, 641-652.

Zinman, B., Vranic, M., Albisser, M., Leibel, B., & Marliss, E. (1979). The role of insulin and the metabolic response to exercise in diabetic man. *Diabetes*, **28**(Suppl.1), 76-81.

Chapter 10

Some Rules and Exceptions in the Response of the Pulmonary System to Muscular Exercise

Jerry A. Dempsey
Kathe G. Henke

Exercise represents the physiologic state that imposes the greatest homeostatic demands on all organ systems, including the pulmonary system. We will briefly examine some of these requirements, the capability of the healthy person to respond to these requirements, and some exceptions in health and in disease states where the homeostatic capabilities of the pulmonary system are comprised.

Some of the critical requirements imposed by exercise and their associated adaptations are shown in Table 1 and Figure 1. Note that the increasing metabolic rate demanded by contracting skeletal muscles dictates that mixed venous blood returning to the lungs undergo progressive O_2 desaturation and rising acidity. Hence, the requirement of the gas exchange system for maintaining isocapnic and normoxic conditions in arterial blood is increased severalfold; yet, the reduced time spent by the desaturated hemoglobin molecule in the pulmonary capillary provides less time for the lung to meet this requirement. Nevertheless, arterial blood gas homeostasis is maintained (see Figure 1) during the steady state of any exercise, regardless of the body position in which the exercise is carried out (Dempsey et al., 1977). At least three, closely interrelated control systems combine forces to ensure that the lung's gas exchange functions are met both adequately and efficiently during exercise—namely, control of exercise hyperpnea, control of mechanical work done by the lung and chest wall, and control of alveolar to arterial gas exchange.

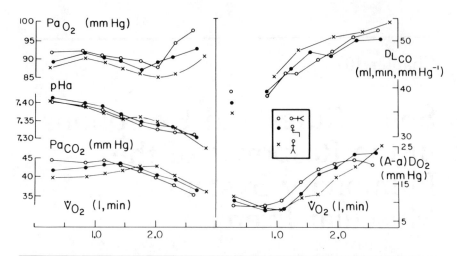

Figure 1 Pulmonary system response to light, moderate, and heavy steady-state exercise in 6 untrained, healthy subjects in the sitting, supine, and standing positions. Note (left panel) the maintenance of arterial PO_2 throughout exercise, the fairly tight control over arterial PCO_2 in mild through moderate exercise, and the hyperventilatory response to the metabolic acidemia of heavy exercise. Diffusion capacity of the lung (DLCO) and the alveolar to arterial PO_2 difference (A-aDO_2) increase during exercise; though they are posture-dependent at rest, they show no differences during heavy exercise, probably because the pulmonary capillary blood volume expands to a similar extent in both postures. *Note.* From "Pulmonary Adaptation to Exercise: Effects of Exercise Type and Duration, Chronic Hypoxia, and Physical Training" by J.A. Dempsey et al., 1977, *Annals of the New York Academy of Science,* **301,** p. 245. Copyright 1977 by the New York Academy of Science. Reprinted by permission.

Rules

Over a wide range of mild through moderate steady state exercise, the ventilatory response is fairly proportional to the change in CO_2 production. There are some departures from this rule, and indeed a wide range of responses may be found among healthy individuals, but rarely does the arterial PCO_2 deviate more than $\pm$ 3-5 mmHg from the resting level (Dempsey, Mitchell, & Smith, 1984). Although the mechanisms controlling this ventilatory response are highly controversial and remain unknown (Dempsey, Vidruk, & Mastenbrook, 1980; Dempsey, Vidruk, & Mitchell, 1980; Whipp, 1981) it is safe to conclude at this point that the response contains at least three elements and/or mechanisms. First, a primary "feed-forward" drive to breathe must occur coincident with locomotion (i.e., a so-called neurogenic stimulus from working limbs or the locomotor cortex) or secondary to increasing CO_2 by working skele-

Table 1   Requirements and Responses in the Healthy Pulmonary Control System During Exercise

Pulmonary Variables Affected by Exercise	Rest	Moderate Exercise	Heavy Exercise	Units
$\dot{V}O_2 \sim \dot{V}CO_2$	0.3	1	3	l/min
Mixed venous $-$ O_2 content	15	11	6	ml O_2, 100 ml
$-PCO_2$	46	52	65	mmHg
Alveolar ventilation	5	25	140	l/min
Pulmonary blood flow	5	11	20	l/min
Pul. art. pressure	15	20	25	mmHg
Left atrial pressure	5	6	8	mmHg
Pul. vascular resistance	150	125	100	dynes•sec^{-1}•
Pul. capillary blood vol.	70	125	200	ml^{-5}

tal muscles (i.e., some mechanism linked to the enhanced blood flow or transport of CO_2 back to the lung) (Dempsey et al., 1985; Whipp, 1981).

This so-called primary mechanism is not sufficient by itself, however, to provide the homeostasis of arterial PCO_2 shown in Figure 1. This homeostasis requires secondary chemoreceptor feedback mechanisms capable of sensing and responding to relatively small "errors" in arterial and cerebral fluid acid-base status. The incorporation of these feedback elements in the control system are important when the proportional increase in the feed-forward stimulus with exercise is not *exactly* proportional to the increase in metabolic rate (Dempsey et al., 1985).

The third element in this ventilatory control system is concerned with how each breath is taken, i.e., the frequency, the depth, the time of inspiration, time of expiration, pause between breaths, the lung volume from which each breath is initiated, etc. These response characteristics are probably under purposeful control. For example, it would not make sense in terms of mechanical efficiency if the increase in ventilation was accomplished solely by an increasing frequency of breathing, or if the depth of each breath was increased solely by encroaching on the expiratory side of the resting lung volume, or if the timing of the breath was such that the time for inspiration was 90% (rather than the usual 50% or less) of the total time to take each breath. Accordingly, receptors in the respiratory muscles of the chest wall and in the airways and parenchyma are plentifully equipped with sensory pathways to respiratory center neurons, the higher central nervous system (CNS), and segmentally to the spinal cord. This mechanical feedback system is highly sensitive to inappropriate changes in pressures developed in the thorax, to the intrinsic length/tension and force/velocity characteristics of the respiratory muscles, and to the mechanical status of the lung and airways. Thus, during exercise a fairly well-maintained resting lung volume, coupled with the combination of increasing frequency and tidal volume, are such that resistance and compliance of the lung remain fairly constant despite the very high tidal volumes achieved in heavy exercise (Dempsey et al., 1980). Even when extra homeostatic requirements are superimposed on exercise, such as the metabolic acidosis of increased lactic acid production in very heavy exercise, the ventilatory control system responds by increasing ventilation out of proportion to increasing CO_2 production. The resulting hypocapnia provides partial compensation for a progressive metabolic acidosis.

The Respiratory Muscles

Respiratory muscles ensure the highly efficient transformation of inspiratory neural drive into pressure generation within the thorax. It is unlikely that the respiratory muscles ever actually fatigue during exercise. These "essential" skeletal muscles are probably protected from fatigue in a number of ways (Dempsey & Fregosi, 1985; Fixler, Atkins, Mitchell, & Horwitz, 1976; Rochester & Briscoe, 1979): (a) More than just the diaphragm is available to generate inspiratory efforts during exercise. Accessory intercostal muscles come into play even in relatively moderate exercise; in heavy exercise other accessory muscles, even those of the neck and upper back, assist in the development of a negative inspiratory pleural pressure. (b) The metabolic capacity of inspiratory muscles, especially the diaphragm, far exceeds that of limb locomotor muscles of similar fiber type and is more like cardiac muscle in this respect. (c) Functionally the diaphragm is placed in a mechanically advantageous position; active expiration causes an increased abdominal pressure, thereby pushing the diaphragm to a greater length, capable of generating more pressure on the subsequent inspiration. (d) The blood flow and therefore oxygen transport to the diaphragm is greatly enhanced during exercise, for the inspiratory muscles share in an even greater proportion of the total increase in cardiac output than do limb locomotor muscles.

The results of these characteristics and adaptations of the respiratory muscles are that glycogen is spared and fat is preferentially metabolized even during rather heavy exercise. The pressures developed across the diaphragm even in very heavy exercise do not approach the maximum pressures the diaphragm is capable of developing (at rest) or maintaining for very long periods. Finally, more recent evidence points to an important role for recruitment of muscles outside the thorax (England & Bartlett, 1982). The hyperpnea of exercise is accompanied by abduction of the laryngeal musculature, which increases the diameter of the extrathoracic upper airway at a location that presents the major resistance to airflow. This would, of course, reduce the resistive load presented to the respiratory muscles. This compensation is aided further by dilation of bronchiolar smooth muscle and the redirection of airflow from primarily nasal to lower resistance oral routes.

The Lungs

The morphological characteristics and the adaptability of the lung itself seem ideally suited to the exercising state. Note in Figure 1 that even though the alveolar to arterial PO_2 difference does widen about threefold in heavy exercise, alveolar PO_2 increases sufficiently, so that the arterial PO_2 remains very close to resting values. Certainly a critical characteristic of the lung that enhances oxygen transport is its architecture, i.e., the 140 m^2 alveolar capillary surface area and an extremely thin (only a few microns thick) air-blood barrier (Weibel, 1983) (see Figure 2).

In addition to these morphological characteristics, a key adaptation to exercise is the threefold expansion of the pulmonary capillary bed, which is achieved primarily by recruitment of capillaries that were unperfused in the resting state. The time spent by a red cell in the pulmonary capillary is determined by the ratio of pulmonary blood flow to pulmonary capillary blood volume. If the pulmonary capillary bed were incapable of expanding substantially during exercise (see Table 1 and Figure 2), the transit time of the red cell in the pulmonary capillaries would be reduced to less than one-quarter its time at rest, and diffusion equilibrium of alveolar gas with pulmonary capillary blood would not occur by the time the blood reached the end of the pulmonary capillary (Johnson, Taylor, & Larson, 1965). The diffusion pathway is also closely protected during exercise by the substantial lymphatic drainage of the interstitial fluid space in the lung. This protects against fluid accumulation in the interstitial or alveolar spaces, in the face of very high pulmonary blood flows and high turnover of lung water.

These, then, are the qualities and characteristics of the control of breathing, the control of lung and chest wall mechanics, and the regulation of the lung's gas exchange that ensure an efficient homeostasis of arterial blood gases and acid-base status during exercise.

Exceptions to the Homeostatic Efficient Response: Some Examples in Health

Now we will turn to some of the exceptions to these "rules," where—in the super-healthy, or under various types of environmental stresses, or in certain disease states—homeostasis is not maintained either because

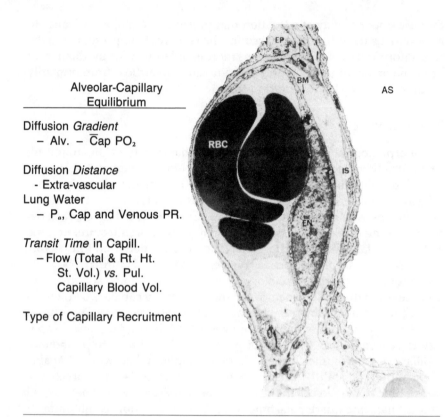

Alveolar-Capillary
Equilibrium

Diffusion *Gradient*
– Alv. – $\overline{C}$ap PO_2

Diffusion *Distance*
- Extra-vascular
Lung Water
– P_a, Cap and Venous PR.

Transit Time in Capill.
– Flow (Total & Rt. Ht.
St. Vol.) *vs.* Pul.
Capillary Blood Vol.

Type of Capillary Recruitment

Figure 2 The alveolar capacity diffusion pathway and the determinants of alveolar-capillary equilibrium. AS = alveolar space, IS = interstitial fluid space, BM = basement membrane, EP = alveolar epithelium, EN = endothelial cell, and RBC = red blood cell. (Also see Table 1 and Figure 4.)

gas exchange is inadequate or, most importantly, because the physiological cost of maintaining or attempting to maintain homeostasis is too high.

Time-Dependent Tachypnea in Endurance Exercise

Heavy, prolonged endurance exercise is commonly characterized by an inability of many organ systems to maintain a steady-state response. This is particularly true if the exercise is carried out in a hot environment (Dempsey et al., 1977; Hanson, Claremont, Dempsey, & Reddan, 1982). A well-known marker of an unstable response in these conditions is the occurrence of a time-dependent "cardiovascular drift," as shown by increasing tachycardia, rising cardiac output, and a competitive redistribution of blood flow among skin versus working locomotor muscles versus the essential organs.

The pulmonary system is not an exception to this inability to maintain steady-state conditions. Thus, even under the carefully controlled enviromental conditions of the laboratory, minute ventilation increases over time at a constant heavy work load secondary to an increased breathing frequency, and a respiratory alkalosis commonly prevails. This non-homeostatic, inefficient response is particularly marked in a hot environment (Hanson et al., 1982). Under these conditions, the increase in breathing frequency becomes very marked as the race progresses, resulting in an increase in dead space ventilation to the point where overall minute ventilation increases markedly with little or no change in arterial PCO_2.

This highly inefficient, time-dependent increase in wasted ventilation is the antithesis of the usual concept of a falling ratio of dead space to tidal volume during short-term exercise. The increasing breathing frequency is also a unique response in that most ventilatory stimuli in healthy humans primarily cause an increase in tidal volume. Mediation of this time-dependent tachypnea may be through gradually increasing core and blood temperatures (which affect both the carotid body and probably higher CNS receptors concerned with temperature regulation). Indeed, when the body surface is continually cooled experimentally, and much of the rise in core temperature during heavy prolonged exercise is prevented, this also prevents most of the hyperventilation. Perhaps then we are dealing here with a vestigial remnant of the panting response so prevalent in and important to animals such as the dog for regulation of brain temperature. However, we can think of no real useful purpose served by the human's tachypneic response in long-term exercise, which appears to result only in an inefficient gas exchange and a marked discomfort in the act of breathing.

Exercise-Induced Arterial Hypoxemia in Very Heavy Exercise

Even though arterial PO_2 is maintained at resting levels in heavy exercise up to 3-4 1/min $\dot{V}O_2$ (Figure 1, Table 1), the fact that the lung is not a perfect gas exchanger under these conditions is indicated by the finding that arterial PO_2 does not rise coincident with the increasing alveolar PO_2, i.e., a widened alveolar-arterial PO_2 difference prevails. We are also reminded that the ventilatory control system's response to heavy exercise is an imperfect one. A substantial hyperventilation occurs with increasing metabolic acidosis, but this compensatory response is incomplete, for arterial pH is reduced significantly below resting levels. More recently we have observed what we consider to be "failure" in both the gas exchange and ventilatory control capabilities of the pulmonary system dur-

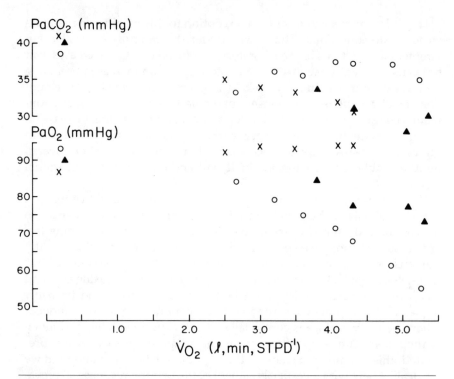

Figure 3 Effects of progressive exercise to very heavy loads on arterial blood gases in 3 representative, very highly trained runners. Hypoxemia was most evident in the runners who showed a combination of no or little alveolar hyperventilaion (PaCO₂ 35-40 mmHg) combined with an excessively wide alveolar to arterial PO₂ difference (35-45 mmHg).

ing the performance of extremely heavy exercise in highly trained individuals (Dempsey, Hanson, & Henderson, 1984). Some examples during treadmill running are shown in Figure 3. Note the contrast among the three athletes depicted in this figure. In one subject (X), arterial PO_2 is maintained with increasing exercise load, i.e., the usual concept. The other two examples show varying degrees of moderate to rather severe arterial hypoxemia as $\dot{V}O_2$ increases in excess of 3.5-4 1/minute. This pattern was evident in more than half of the 16 highly trained athletes studied (Dempsey, Hanson, & Henderson, 1984).

What causes this hypoxemia? First, the degree of hyperventilation in these athletes is inadequate in the sense that, given the extremely high metabolic demand ($\dot{V}O_2 > 5$ 1/min), they are unable (or "unwilling") to increase ventilation sufficiently (> 180 1/min V_E) to allow alveolar PO_2 to rise to the usual 115-125 mmHg and $PaCO_2$ to fall to < 30 mmHg. Less well-trained individuals with much lower max $\dot{V}CO_2$ and $\dot{V}O_2$ require substantially lower ventilatory values to achieve these levels of alveolar PO_2

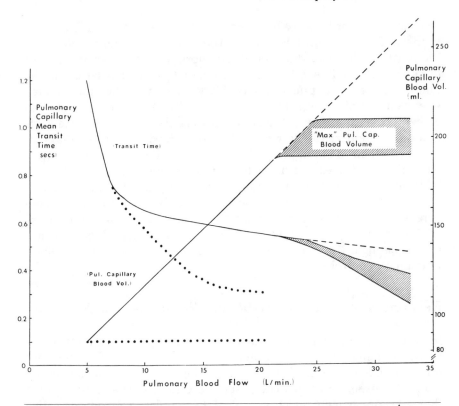

Figure 4   Schematic showing relationship of pulmonary blood flow (Q̇c) to pulmonary capillary blood volume (Vc), to average red cell transit time in the pulmonary capillary. Note in the untrained subject with V̇O₂ max of ~ 3.5 l min and max cardiac output of 20 l/min, Vc increases linearly with Q̇c as exercise increases, and mean red cell transit time is reduced to 0.5-0.6 secs, which is more than adequate to ensure alveolar-end–pulmonary-capillary O₂ equilibrium. Also note the importance of the increasing pulmonary capillary blood volume in the subjects, because if Vc is not able to increase during exercise (...), red cell transit time would fall precipitously as Q̇c increased. This is the problem facing the emphysematous patient with a restricted pulmonary vascular bed. Yet, this may also explain exercise-induced hypoxemia in the athlete at very high work loads, because Vc reaches a maximum expansion at a time when Q̇c continues to increase, thereby markedly shortening transit time. At Q̇c > 24 l/min, contrast the transit time under conditions where Vc might theoretically continue to increase linearly with increasing Q̇c (---), versus more realistic conditions where Vc max is achieved as Q̇c continues to rise (///).

and arterial PCO_2 (see Figure 1 examples). We believe this absence of sufficient hyperventilation in very heavy exercise is attributable to the fact that mechanical limitations are being approached by the high flow rates achieved in these endurance athletes (Dempsey, Hanson, & Henderson, 1984; Dempsey, Vidruk, & Mitchell, 1985).

A second major cause of hypoxemia was the extremely wide alveolar to arterial PO_2 difference (35-45 mmHg) achieved at these high work loads. We attribute this to a diffusion disequilibrium, that is, an inability of desaturated mixed venous blood to equilibrate with alveolar gas in the time available in the pulmonary capillary. Why does this time become so exceedingly short, less than .3-.4 seconds? The key here, as mentioned earlier, is the expansion of the pulmonary capillary bed. It is conceivable that the pulmonary capillary bed achieves its maximum at a cardiac output of less than 25 l/min, that is, $\dot{V}O_2 \sim 4$ l/m, and that when pulmonary blood flow continues to increase further in persons with very high metabolic demands and high maximum cardiac outputs, the transit time of the red cell in the pulmonary capillary simply becomes too short to ensure diffusion equilibrium with alveolar gas (see Figure 4). Thus, as incredible as it may seem, these data suggest that many athletes capable of completing a 4-minute mile are doing so in the present of a "failing" pulmonary control system.

Responses to Non-Steady-State, Transient-Type Exercise

Inefficiency and inability to achieve homeostasis in the pulmonary system are not limited to heavy or prolonged exercise in athletic events, but occur commonly in everyday events requiring an increased metabolic demand. For example, immediate onset of exertion, such as running up a flight of stairs, usually results in a lag of the ventilatory response relative to the increased metabolic demand. Thus, a transient hypoxemia will prevail until a steady state is reached and the sluggish rise in V_E matches $\dot{V}CO_2$.

Numerous examples also occur in the industrial setting. Work accomplished with small muscle groups, e.g., the arms, almost always requires a greater ventilatory (and higher breathing frequency) response than does work with larger muscle groups. Changes in posture during the work task also lead to a change in the length of the various respiratory muscles, which in turn require compensation on the part of these muscles in order to maintain ventilation. In our analysis of assembly line workers completing manual tasks requiring 3-4 minutes of time per task (e.g., building an automobile tire), we found that the ventilatory and heart rate responses never achieved a steady state, but were constantly changing, even though task completion required an average energy operative which was only 30-40% of $\dot{V}O_2$ max (Reddan, Dempsey, doPico, & Rankin, 1974). Further, over the course of the day it was not uncommon to see ventilatory and cardiovascular "drift" analogous to that seen at much heavier prolonged work loads in the trained athlete (see above). This was especially true if the workplace was hot.

Our point of emphasis here is not that the pulmonary system is incapable of maintaining homeostasis and an efficient response during moderate to heavy exercise. Rather, we wish to clarify that the responses shown in the strictly controlled laboratory environment may bear little resemblance to the more demanding complexities of work in the real world.

Short-Term Adaptation in a Hypoxic Environment

The pulmonary system as the first line of defense for gas transport is severely taxed when normal human subjects sojourn at high altitudes. At moderate altitudes, around 10,000-12,000 feet, the pulmonary response is adequate in terms of gas exchange, but the physiological cost is high. Thus, one sees in the exercising sojourner at this altitude a marked hyperventilation with $PaCO_2$ ~ 20-25 mmHg, high breathing frequency, and a very high work of breathing secondary to increased flow resistance (Dempsey et al., 1977; Thoden et al., 1969). These levels of hypocapnia are also sensed in the CNS, and cerebral blood flow will often be markedly reduced as the brain sacrifices O_2 transport in an attempt to protect its PCO_2 and acid-base status (Dempsey et al., 1977; Dempsey, Thomson, Alexander, Forster, & Chosy, 1975). On the other hand, arterial PO_2 is maintained from rest to heavy exercise to within 10 mmHg of resting levels; with the increase of red cell production and hemoglobin concentration after 2 weeks at this altitude, one may even see a normal arterial oxygen content in the exercising sojourner. Thus, at this altitude in the healthy sojourner, the major problem of gas transport during exercise is with the reduced stroke volume and cardiac output at any given exercise load (Dempsey, Thomson, Forster, Cerny, & Chosy, 1975).

The primary problem, then, with the pulmonary response at high altitudes is its physiological cost in terms of exertional dyspnea and the work of breathing. If the sea-level native sojourns at even higher altitudes approaching 14,000-15,000 feet, arterial PO_2 would be on the extremely steep portion of the HbO_2 dissociation curve, and diffusion limitation would occur even in moderate exercise (Dempsey et al., 1977). Hyperventilation, especially during exercise, is even more extreme at this altitude ($PaCO_2$ ~ 15-17 mmHg); but in this case this high ventilatory cost does not prevent O_2 desaturation in arterial blood, which falls precipitously even in moderate exercise.

If the sojourner chooses to go to the ultimate—i.e., to the peak of Everest—and forgets his supplemental oxygen, then the true limits of the pulmonary response to exercise are probably achieved, for arterial PO_2 is now in the 25 mmHg range and falls precipitously even in very mild exercise (West, 1984). From the ventilatory standpoint, no exercise is "mild," because each step requires about four or five huge, near-vital-capacity size breaths, and even resting PCO_2 is less than 10 mmHg. Clearly, both the ventilatory cost and the arterial hypoxemia become limiting factors in exercise under these extreme conditions. The recent conquering of Everest without supplemental O_2 has been hailed as evidence of a remarkable physiological tolerance in the healthy human—but perhaps a "winner" here shouldn't be proclaimed until all of the chronic aftereffects of these brief bouts with anoxia have been assessed.

Implications for Physical Training in Healthy Persons

The findings in a number of examples cited above are that the lung can't keep up with the metabolic demands of the locomotor muscles. This implies that as widespread as the morphological effects of physical training might be in the body, the pulmonary system may be largely left out of this adaptive process. Perhaps the physical training stimulus or the trained state increases aerobic capacity primarily through its effects on factors intrinsic and extrinsic to the heart that control cardiac function (max cardiac output), on the systemic vasculature (skeletal muscle capillary density), and on the metabolic capacity of locomotor muscles. The lung parenchyma, airways, and capillary blood volume—perhaps in some respects even the chest wall—remain relatively untouched via the physical training process!

Thus the pulmonary control system is no longer able to match the demands imposed by other truly adapted organ systems, and arterial blood gas homeostasis is sacrificed. The data available on the relative effects of chronic physical training on the various organ systems tend to support this hypothesis. For example, physical training in animals has been shown to increase mitochondrial enzyme activity in locomotor muscle approximately 25-50%, whereas the diaphragm in these same animals undergoes either no discernible adaptation or one that is less than a third of that in locomotor muscles of similar fiber type (Dempsey & Fregosi, 1984; Moore & Gollnick, 1982). Similarly, and to an even greater extent, the gas exchange apparatus seems to be immune to the intermittent training stimulus, because the number and size of alveoli, size of the pulmonary vascular bed, total gas exchange surface area, and diffusion capacity of the lung at rest or exercise all undergo no change with chronic physical training in animals or humans (Dempsey & Fregosi, 1984; Dempsey et al., 1977). Furthermore, the human athlete does not have a greater diffusion capacity than the nonathlete. Even chronic physical training at high altitude, which significantly increases work capacity in sedentary humans, has no effect on gas exchange characteristics of the lung (Dempsey et al., 1977).

These negative data do not imply that the lung or the chest wall are incapable of adaptation through more specific or more truly chronic, sustained stimuli than is offered by intermittent physical training. There are several examples of true adaptation in the pulmonary system. Truly *chronic* hypoxia (such as found in natives of high altitudes) dramatically increases the gas exchange surface area of the lung. Secondly, normal individuals who specifically train their breathing muscles can increase both the power and endurance of their ventilatory efforts, and the animal whose airway resistance is markedly and permanently elevated (via tracheal banding) shows increased metabolic capacity of his diaphragm in response to this severe increase in the chronic ventilatory load. Finally, even the emphysematous patient with hyperinflated lungs undergoes adaptation in his short, flattened diaphragm, so that greater tension (or force) may be exerted during inspiration at a shorter muscle length.

At one time we believed that the absence of physical training effects on the pulmonary system could be explained by the fact that the reserve of the lung and the respiratory muscles were more than would ever be required in the exercising state, regardless of the load demanded (Dempsey & Rankin, 1977). More recent findings indicate that this explanation is no longer adequate, and that indeed there are circumstances where these apparent reserves of the pulmonary system are eroded by the process of physical training. Thus, as fitness increases, the margin of safety is reduced between maximum O_2 consumption achievable by the body and the pulmonary system's ability to transport O_2 from alveolar air to arterial blood.

Special Problems Presented by the Exercising Patient With Chronic Lung Disease

The response to exercise of any intensity in the patient with chronic obstructive or restrictive lung disease is the antithesis of that enjoyed by the healthy individual. In general, the problem in disease states is the erosion of the functional reserve capacities of the lung and chest wall. The result is an extremely low exercise capacity, which is symptom-limited by extreme shortness of breath and is often accompanied by inadequate gas exchange, abnormal breathing patterns, and abnormal coordination of respiratory muscles. We provide just a few examples of some of these problems here and refer the reader to more extensive discussions of the exercise response in various pulmonary diseases (Killian & Campbell, 1983; Sharp, 1984; Wasserman & Whipp, 1975).

Control of Ventilation During Exercise

The basic problem with ventilatory control during exercise in these patients is that disease state superimposes additional stimuli and/or inhibitions on the normally existent primary drives to exercise hyperpnea. These influences often conflict. For example, the increasing inspiratory drive coincident with increasing exercise levels is inhibited by an increased airway resistance; and if hypoxemia and/or acidemia accompanies the exercise (see below), then an even greater disparity between inspiratory drive (or "effort") and ventilatory output ensues. The greater this neuro-mechanical, input/output disparity, the greater the dyspnea, for the patient's ventilatory control system is forced to make choices between preserving arterial blood chemistry versus minimizing his work to breathe. The combination of asphyxia (even small amounts of hypoxemia plus CO_2 retention) with elevated airway resistance produces profound anxiety, and every breath becomes an almost purely volitionally controlled event. Obviously, then, accomplishing a breath becomes a higher priority than completing (or often perhaps even starting) an exercise task.

The regulation of breathing pattern also, in addition to total minute ventilation, is characterized by the effects of overriding and opposing influences. For example, patients with predominantly large airway obstructive disease would attempt to keep frequency low and patients with predominantly parenchymal lung disease would try to minimize an increase in tidal volume, because in each case an attempt is made to maintain a mimimal work of breathing while at the same time provide adequate increases in alveolar ventilation. These would be the compensatory responses obtained in the healthy individual who is made for a few minutes to breath through a resister or to be subjected to chest wall strapping. However, these compensations may well be overridden in these patients during exercise, when airway or parenchymal receptors are stimulated, causing a powerful, vagally mediated tachypnea. For example, heart failure and pulmonary congestion leading to increased pressures in the pulmonary arteries, veins, and the interstitial fluid spaces of the lung (especially during exercise when pulmonary blood flow is increased) give rise to tachypnea (Wilson & Ferrara, 1983). Another common associated occurrence in these patients is an erratic breathing pattern as large breath-to-breath fluctuations occur in the frequency, tidal volume, and ratio of inspiratory time to total breath time (Ti/Ttot). This inability to maintain the steady-state response to any sort of prolonged exercise (sometimes as short as 5 minutes) applies to most cardiopulmonary responses in pulmonary disease patients. This contrasts markedly with the healthy person, who shows no significant departure from the steady-state response until work is very hard and very prolonged (see above).

The COPD patient with severe hyperinflation also has a short, flat, diaphragm, which places this major inspiratory muscle at a substantial mechanical disadvantage, i.e., the diaphragm's capability as a force or tension generator is greatly compromised (Sharp, 1984). Thus, the patient comes to rely more and more on accessory respiratory muscles for inspiration. This happens especially during exercise, when inspiratory drive is high and where the shortened times available for expiration may cause even further hyperinflation and thus a greater diaphragmatic shortening prior to the initiation of inspiration. The diaphragm and other respiratory muscles may be further compromised if O_2 transport to these muscles is reduced by either arterial hypoxemia or reduced cardiac output.

All of these factors place the respiratory muscles in a precarious, fatigue-susceptible position. Accordingly, even mild exercise causes near-maximal activation of all accessory inspiratory muscles in the rib cage, neck, and upper back, at substantial volitional effort and metabolic cost. Each expiration also requires activation of abdominal and intercostal expiratory muscles in an attempt to complete expiration in the short time allotted. This marked activation of expiratory muscles is important in two ways for completing the subsequent inspiration: (a) It prevents further shortening of the diaphragm and other inspiratory muscles, which are thus better tension generators; and (b) when abdominal muscles suddenly relax at end expiration, the abdominal pressure now swings in a negative direction as the abdominal cavity expands; to the extent that this pressure change is reflected in the pleural space, lung inflation during inspiration will be accomplished passively, i.e., largely as the consequence of the energy expended during the preceding expiration.

Gas Exchange During Exercise

Exercise-induced hypoxemia is, of course, a major concern in the patient with chronic lung disease, because as mixed venous O_2 content falls and the velocity of pulmonary blood flow increases with exercise (Table 1), the ability to ensure maintained arterial oxygenation becomes critically dependent upon (a) a marked increase in alveolar ventilation that is out of proportion to increased pulmonary blood flow (i.e., high overall $\dot{V}A:\dot{Q}c$ ratios); (b) a closely maintained, very narrow distribution of alveolar ventilation to perfusion ratios throughout the lung; and (c) sufficient time in the pulmonary capillary, coupled with a diffusion capacity that is adequate to ensure alveolar-end pulmonary capillary O_2 equilibrium.

The fact that arterial hypoxemia is commonly observed in the exercising patient—even in cases where hypoxemia is absent or only borderline at rest—is attributable to the disease process with one or more of these critical adaptations. For example, inadequate response of alveolar ventilation with increasing CO_2 production commonly occurs because of a mechanical limitation to airflow due either to increased airway resistance or to an increase in dead space ventilation secondary to an extreme tachypnic breathing pattern. Incomplete diffusion equilibrium may occur during exercise secondary to inadequate equilibration time in cases in which the emphysema patient is unable to adequately expand his pulmonary vascular bed in the face of a normally rising pulmonary blood flow. Even only a relatively small right to left shunt (of ~ < 10-15% of pulmonary blood flow) existing in the lung becomes an important cause of hypoxemia when mixed venous O_2 content is reduced during exercise.

Pulmonary Vasculature

The pulmonary vascular system and hemodynamics may be severely compromised in the patient with chronic obstructive pulmonary disease and may be worsened with exercise. This should be an important consideration in exercising these individuals. During exercise in healthy individuals, mean pulmonary artery pressure (P$\overline{p}$a) will increase from a resting value of approximately 10 mmHg to about 25 mmHg, seldom exceeding 30 mmHg. This increase is due to the increased cardiac output during exercise. The pulmonary capillary bed expands by recruiting previously unperfused capillaries to accommodate this increased flow, so that pulmonary vascular resistance falls.

The individual with COPD often has elevated P$\overline{p}$a at rest, commonly accompanied by hypertrophied pulmonary arteriolar smooth muscle. P$\overline{p}$a has been shown to increase abnormally during even modest levels of exercise in these patients (1.5-2 METs) (Brown & Wasserman, 1981; Horsfield, Segal, & Bishop, 1968; Kitchin, Lowther, & Matthews, 1961; Light, Mintz, Linden, & Brown, 1984; Wright et al, 1983), and values in excess of 70 mmHg have been reported (see Table 2). Pulmonary vascular

Table 2   Effects of Exercise on the Pulmonary Vasculature and Arterial PO_2

Pulmonary Functions (unit)	Subject Status	Rest Air	Exercise (2 METs) Air	O_2
Mean pulmonary artery pressure	NL	18	23	
(mmHg)	COPD	28	45	39
Pulmonary vascular resistance	NL	100	75	
(dynes•sec^{-1}•cm^{-5})	COPD	250	275	220
PaO_2	NL	90	90	
(mmHg)	COPD	60	55	446

resistance (PVR) is also markedly elevated in many patients with COPD; during exercise PVR does not decrease as in normals and may even increase in some (see Table 2).

There are two major explanations for these findings: (a) destruction of the pulmonary vascular bed and (b) hypoxic pulmonary vasoconstriction. Destruction of the pulmonary vascular bed makes it incapable of expanding sufficiently to accommodate the increased blood flow during exercise, so that P͞p͞a and PVR are elevated far above normal. Alveolar hypoxia is a major cause of pulmonary vasoconstriction. In many patients— especially those who underventilate—exercise increases pulmonary arteriolar vasoconstriction at a time when pulmonary blood flow is increasing in an already stiff vascular bed. Interstitial edema, which could in time occlude even more vessels, may result in some extreme instances.

These changes can also affect hemodynamic performance. Although cardiac index (cardiac output/body surface area) is reported to be normal in most patients at rest and during exercise (Brown & Wasserman, 1981; Light et al., 1984; Olvey, Reduto, Stevens, Deaton, & Miller, 1980), tachycardia is a general finding. Stroke volume, then, is likely to be diminished (Light et al., 1980). Olvey et al. (1980) report that, in general, left ventricular function is normal in patients with severe COPD; right ventricular function, as measured by right ventricular ejection fraction (RVEF), however, is often abnormal in these patients (RVEF < 50%). Not only was RVEF abnormal at rest, but it failed to increase during exercise. Normal healthy subjects increase RVEF (67% at rest to 80% during exercise), whereas the patients with COPD showed no change.

Not all individuals with COPD demonstrate abnormal response to exercise. What causes these individual differences? Patients who are hypoxic at rest and those with marked destruction of their pulmonary capillaries are at greater risk for developing pulmonary hypertension during exercise. Kitchen et al. (1961) found that in patients with emphysema, those with a low or normal alveolar ventilation were hypoxemic and had pulmonary hypertension, whereas those with high resting ventilation had normal or near normal oxygen saturation and little pulmonary hypertension.

Supplemental oxygen can, potentially, reverse pulmonary vasoconstriction. In a healthy person at a high altitude, for example, alveolar hypoxia causes pulmonary vasoconstriction and, consequently, increased P͞p͞a and PVR. Oxygen administration completely reverses this. This is not the case in the person with chronic lung disease. The degenerative process of emphysema irreversibly destroys portions of the pulmonary vascular bed, and arteriolar smooth muscle hypertrophies. The administration of oxygen, while alleviating pulmonary vasoconstriction, can do nothing to lessen the increased resistance of the now noncompliant pulmonary vascular bed. Although oxygen administration during exercise can decrease P͞p͞a and PVR and increase RVEF, these improvements are modest (Brown

& Wasserman, 1981; Horsfield et al., 1968; Kitchen et al, 1961; Light et al., 1984; Olvey et al., 1980; Wright et al., 1983).

The data presented here suggest that the cardiovascular system of individuals with COPD may be compromised during exercise by increased $P\bar{p}a$ and PVR, and by a low RVEF. The benefits of exercise should be weighed with these potential hazards in exercising the patient with COPD. Supplemental oxygen during exercise in some patients with moderate to severe disease may lessen these risks.

Exercise Training in the Patient With Pulmonary Disease

Exercise is often an integral part of the rehabilitation program of a pulmonary patient. What then are the long-term effects of exercise for these individuals (Table 3)? Most studies report increases in exercise tolerance, usually measured as increased time to exhaustion or increased exercise workload (Belman & Rendregan, 1982; Brown & Wasserman, 1981; Hale, Cumming, & Spriggs, 1978). Some studies report increases in symptom-limited $\dot{V}O_2$ max (Hale et al, 1978; Orenstein et al., 1981; Sergysels, De Coston, Degre, & Denolen, 1979).

There are several problems in interpreting the results of these studies, though. First, persons with lung disease rarely reach true $\dot{V}O_2$ "max," because ventilatory limits are reached first. This makes it difficult to determine if improvements are from actual changes or only from increased effort. Second, there is little clear evidence for the peripheral or

Table 3   Chronic Effects of Exercise in Individuals With Chronic Lung Disease

Function	Training Effects (2 Mos.-2 Yrs.)
Exercise tolerance	↑
Hemodynamic and peripheral blood lactate, heart rate stroke volume, cardiac output	→
Pulmonary function	→
Arterial PO_2	↑→ Rest, → Exercise
Arterial PCO_2	→ Rest
Mean pulmonary artery pressure	↓? Rest, → Exercise
Respiratory muscle function	↑?
Dyspnea	↓
Supplemental O_2	↑?

hemodynamic adaptation that would accompany a true increase in $\dot{V}O_2$ max. Belman and Wasserman (1981) found no change in mitochondrial enzymes following training in patients with COPD. Other studies reported no changes in blood lactate levels following training. Hale et al. (1978) add that the Hawthorne effect and improved psychological factors also affect performance on exercise tests. Finally, adults with COPD are very detrained, sedentary or bedridden, and often malnourished. It is felt that they cannot exercise at intensities sufficient for training to occur. On the other hand, Orenstein and co-workers (1981) found changes after training indicating increases in $\dot{V}O_2$ max in their patients with cystic fibrosis. This group was generally more active and certainly younger than most adults with COPD that have been studied, though, and were able to work at higher intensitites.

Although there have been some anecdotal changes reported in pulmonary function with physical training, there is a lack of evidence of any significant changes in spirometry, lung volumes, compliance, airway resistance, and physiologic dead space (Belman & Wasserman, 1981; Braun, Faulkner, Hughes, Roussos, & Sahgal, 1983). Resting and exercise blood gases also do not change as a result of exercise training.

Exercise training may increase the endurance of the ventilatory muscles. Keens et al. (1977) and Orenstein and co-workers (1981) found increases in maximum sustained ventilatory capacity after exercise training in children and young adults with cystic fibrosis. Belman, however, found no change in ventilatory muscle endurance following exercise training in his subjects. These differences may be explained by the fact that Belman's subjects, who were much older, were not able to attain exercise ventilations sufficient to train the ventilatory muscles. It may be difficult to see an effect of exercise training on the ventilatory muscles for other reasons as well. As previously mentioned, the diaphragm and other inspiratory muscles have high metabolic capacities—they may already be "trained" to a high degree. Studies in which healthy subjects underwent whole body physical training with no effect on ventilatory muscle endurance support this contention. COPD imposes a load on the respiratory system. This is in itself a form of training carried on 24 hours a day. The low levels of exercise achieved by those with COPD may not add enough additional stress to train their respiratory systems to any further extent.

Specific training of the respiratory muscles may improve their endurance. Leith and Bradley (1976) found increases in ventilatory muscle endurance in healthy subjects who specifically trained for endurance. Belman and Mittman (1980) and Pardy, Revengton, Despas, & Macklem (1981) report increases in ventilatory muscle endurance and exercise tolerance in adults with COPD after specific training of the respiratory muscles. This type of training probably imposes a greater load on these muscles than conventional exercise.

Many patients report lessened dyspnea following a program of exercise training. For the most part, this cannot be attributed to any change in stimulus to breathe (hypoxemia or metabolic acidosis). Some relief from dyspnea may be explained by improvement in psychological factors, or some general desensitization to dyspnea (Belman & Wasserman, 1981).

As mentioned previously, $P\bar{p}a$ is elevated at rest and during exercise in patients with COPD. Two studies have reported decreases in $P\bar{p}a$ at rest after exercise training. More research needs to be conducted in this area to determine what changes occur in the pulmonary vascular bed with long-term exercise.

In sum, the effects of long-term exercise in the person with chronic lung disease are unclear. Exercise tolerance improves, but the mechanism for this improvement and the long-term benefits for the patients are unknown.

A Course for Rehabilitation

What then would be a prudent course of rehabilitation? First, patients should be tested to identify those at risk for developing right heart failure during exercise. There is still no reliable way to quantitate pulmonary hypertension by noninvasive techniques. However, there are tests available for identifying the potential for exercise-induced pulmonary hypertension. Simple ear oximetry at rest and during exercise can identify those patients at risk for arterial O_2 desaturation and, thus, for developing pulmonary hypertension via hypoxic vasoconstriction during exercise. An impaired diffusing capacity at rest (and especially one which fails to increase during exercise) can help identify patients with limited dimension of their pulmonary vascular beds, whose $P\bar{p}a$ and PVR may increase dangerously during exercise.

Second, the use of supplemental oxygen during exercise can be an important aid to the rehabilitation program. Current recommendations are for the use of oxygen during exercise for those patients whose resting or exercise PaO_2 is less than 55 mmHg. This may be too liberal an estimate when one considers that (a) the combination of even very mild exercise with a PaO_2 in the 60-70 mmHg range causes a marked increase in ventilatory drive in the healthy person (Dempsey et al., 1977), and (b) hypoxic pulmonary vasoconstriction may occur at alveolar PO_2s in the 65-70 mmHg range, especially under such conditions as exercise where mixed venous PO_2 is reduced (Marshall & Marshall, 1983). Thus, raising PaO_2 to the 70 ± 5 mmHg range by supplemental oxygen would minimize exertional dyspnea and pulmonary hypertension in the COPD patient and also ensure an adequate arterial oxygen content. Indeed, oxygen has been shown to decrease ventilation and dyspnea during exercise in most patients. This may allow patients to exercise longer or to a higher level. The use of oxygen may decrease the abnormally high exercise $P\bar{p}a$ and PVR in patients with COPD. Right ventricular ejection fraction that is abnormally low can be improved with oxygen administration. Of course, it is critical to provide only an appropriate minimum level of arterial oxygenation; thus, different levels of supplementation must be tested by using oximetry at rest *and* at the levels of exercise intended for the training program.

The third consideration is that in severe COPD, respiratory muscle fatigue can occur. Exercising patients in this state can be compared to overtraining athletes. Performance begins to decline, and "use atrophy" develops (Braun et al., 1983). If the athlete then rests until muscles can repair themselves, performance will improve. The patient with severe disease is exercising the respiratory muscles continually; in cases of hyperinflation, these muscles are also placed at a marked mechanic disadvantage. To impose an additional load on a fatigued system may hasten failure of the system. In a study by Braun and Marino (1984) 18 patients were given 5 months of intermittent at-home ventilation therapy. They found significant improvements in vital capacity, MVV, max inspiratory and expiratory pressure, and $PaCO_2$. Patients who had been dyspneic at rest could walk 1 1/2 blocks without dyspnea. It has been suggested that these patients once rested could be given some training or a combination of rest and exercise (Braun et al., 1983). Braun has suggested monitoring fatigue by periodically measuring max mouth pressure of the patients in exercise programs.

With adequate screening, the appropriate administration of oxygen, careful monitoring of fatigue, and a watchful eye on the adequacy of the pulmonary vascular bed, physical training programs may well provide a useful adjunct to a multifaceted treatment program for patients with chronic lung disease.

References

Belman, M.J., & Mittman, C. (1980). Ventilatory muscle training improves exercise capacity in chronic obstructive pulmonary disease patients. *American Review of Respiratory Disease, 121*, 273-280.

Belman, M.J., & Kendregan, B.A. (1982). Physical training fails to improve ventilatory muscle endurance in patients with chronic obstructive pulmonary disease. *Chest, 81*, 440-443.

Belman, M.J., & Wasserman, K. (1981). Exercise training and testing in patients with chronic obstructive pulmonary disease. *Basics of RD, 10*(2), 1-6.

Braun, N.M.T., Faulkner, J., Hughes, R.L., Roussos, D., & Sahgal, V. (1983). When should respiratory muscles be exercised? *Chest*, **84**, 76.

Braun, N.M.T., & Marino, W.D. (1984). Effects of daily intermittent rest of respiratory muscles in patients with severe chronic airflow limitation. *Chest*, **85**(6), 59S.

Brown, H.V., & Wasserman, K. (1981). Exercise performance in chronic obstructive pulmonary disease. *Medical Clinics of North America*, **65**, 525-547.

Brown, H.V., Wasserman, K., & Whipp, B.J. (1977). Strategies of exercise testing in chronic lung disease. *Bulletin Européen Physiopathologie Respiratorie*, **13**, 409-423.

Dempsey, J.A., & Fregosi, R.F. (1985). Adaptability of the pulmonary system to changing metabolic requirements. *American Journal of Cardiology*, **55**, 59D-67D.

Dempsey, J.A., Gledhill, N., Reddan, W.G., Forster, H.V., Hanson, P.G., & Claremont, A.D. (1977). Pulmonary adaptation to exercise: Effects of exercise type and duration, chronic hypoxia, and physical training. *Annals of the New York Academy of Sciences*, **301**, 243.

Dempsey, J.A., Hanson, P., & Henderson, K. (1984). Exercise-induced arterial hypoxemia in healthy humans at sea level. *Journal of Physiology* (London), **335**, 161-175.

Dempsey, J.A., Mitchell, G.S., & Smith, C.A. (1984). Exercise and chemoreception. *American Review of Respiratory Disease*, **129**(Suppl. S31-S34).

Dempsey, J.A., & Rankin, J. (1967). Physiologic adaptations of gas transport systems to muscular exercise in health and disease. *American Journal of Physical Medicine*, **46**, 582-647.

Dempsey, J.A., Thomson, J.M., Alexander, S.C., Forster, H.V., & Chosy, L.W. (1975a). Respiratory influences on acid-base status and their effects on O_2 transport during prolonged muscular work. In H. Howald & J.R. Poortmans (Eds.), *Metabolic adaptation to prolonged exercise; Proceedings of the Second International Symposium on Biochemistry of Exercise* (pp. 56-64). Magglingen, Switzerland.

Dempsey, J.A., Thomson, J.M., Alexander, S.C., Forster, H.V., Cerny, F.C., & Chosy, L.W. (1975b). HbO_2 dissociation in man during prolonged work in chronic hypoxia. *Journal of Applied Physiology*, **38**, 1022-1029.

Dempsey, J.A., Vidruk, E.H., & Mastenbrook, S.M. (1980). Pulmonary control systems in exercise. *Federation Proceedings*, **39**, 1498-1505.

Dempsey, J.A., Vidruk, E.H., & Mitchell, G.S. (1985). Pulmonary control systems in exercise: Update. *Federation Proceedings*, **44**, 2260-2270.

England, S.J., & Bartlett, D. Jr. (1982). Changes in respiratory movements of the human vocal cords during hypernea. *Journal of Applied Physiology*, **52**, 780-785.

Fixler, D.E., Atkins, J.M., Mitchell, J.H., & Horwitz, L.D. (1976). Blood flow to respiratory, cardiac, and limb muscles in dogs during graded exercise. *American Journal of Physiology*, **231**, 1515.

Hale, T., Cumming, G., & Spriggs, J. (1978). The effects of physical training in chronic obstructive pulmonary disease. *Bulletin Européen Physiopathologie Respiratorie*, **14**, 593-608.

Hanson, P., Claremont, A., Dempsey, J., & Reddan, W. (1982). Determinants and consequences of ventilatory responses to competitive endurance running. *Journal of Applied Physiology*, **52**, 615.

Horsfield, K., Segal, N., & Bishop, J.M. (1968). The pulmonary circulation in chronic bronchitis at rest and during exercise breathing air and 80% oxygen. *Clinical Science*, **43**, 473-483.

Johnson, R.L., Taylor, H.F., & Larson, W.H. (1965). Maximal diffusing capacity of the lung for carbon monoxide. *Journal of Clinical Investigation*, **44**, 349-355.

Keens, T.G., Krastins, S.R.B., Wannamaker, E.M., Levison, H., Crozzier, D.H., & Bryan, A.C. (1977). Ventilatory muscle endurance training in normal subjects and patients with cystic fibrosis. *American Review of Respiratory Disease*, **116**, 853-860.

Killian, K.J., & Campbell, E.J. (1983). Dyspnea and exercise. *Annual Review of Physiology*, **45**, 465-479.

Kitchen, A.H., Lowther, C.P., & Matthews, M.B. (1961). The effects of exercise and of breathing oxygen-enriched air on the pulmonary circulation in emphysema. *Clinical Science*, **21**, 93-106.

Leith, D.E., & Bradley, J. (1976). Ventilatory muscle strength and endurance training. *Journal of Applied Physiology*, **41**, 508-516.

Light, R.W., Mintz, H.M., Linden, G.S., & Brown, S.E. (1984). Hemodynamics of patients with severe chronic obstructive pulmonary disease during progressive upright. *American Review of Respiratory Disease*, **130**, 391-395.

Marshall, C., & Marshall, B. (1983). Site and sensitivity for stimulation of hypoxic pulmonary vasoconstriction. *Journal of Applied Physiology: Respiration Environment and Exercise Physiology*, **55**, 711-716.

Moore, R.L., & Gollnick, P.D. (1982). Response of ventilatory muscles of the rat to endurance training. *Pflugers Archive*, **392**, 268-271.

Olvey, S.K., Reduto, L.A., Stevens, P.M., Deaton, W.J., & Miller, R.R. (1980). First pass radionuclide assessment of right and left ventricular ejection fraction in chronic pulmonary disease: Effect of oxygen upon exercise response. *Chest*, **78**, 4-9.

Orenstein, D.M., Franklin, B.A., Doershuk, G.F., Hellerstein, H.F., Germann, K.J., Horowitz, J.G., & Stern, R.C. (1981). Exercise conditioning and cardiopulmonary fitness in cystic fibrosis: The effects of a three-month supervised running program. *Chest*, **80**, 392-398.

Pardy, R.L., Revengton, R.N., Despas, P.J., & Macklem, P.T. (1981). Inspiratory muscle training compared with physiotherapy in patients with chronic airflow limitation. *American Review of Respiratory Disease,* **123,** 426-433.

Reddan, W.G., Dempsey, J.A., doPico, G.A., & Rankin, J. (1974). Pulmonary pathophysiology of industrial disability. In L. Sheving (Ed.), *Chronobiology* (pp. 737-741). Tokyo: Igaku Shoin.

Rochester, D.F., & Briscoe, A.M. (1979). Metabolism of the working diaphragm. *American Review of Respiratory Disease,* **119**(2), 101-106.

Sergysels, R., De Coston, A., Degre, S., & Denolen, H. (1979). Functional evaluation of a physical rehabilitation program including breathing exercises and bicycle training in chronic obstructive lung disease. *Respiration,* **38,** 105-111.

Sharp, J.T. (1984). How diaphragm disorders affect your COPD patients. *Journal of Respiratory Disease,* **5,** 32.

Thoden, J.S., Dempsey, J.A., Redden, W.G., Birnbaum, M.L., Forster, H.V., Grover, H.F., & Rankin, J. (1969). Ventilatory work during steady-state response to exercise. *Federation Proceedings,* **28,** 1316-1321.

Wasserman, K., & Whipp, B.J. (1975). Exercise physiology in health and disease. *American Review of Respiratory Diseases,* **112,** 219-249.

Weibel, E.R. (1983). Is the lung built reasonably? *American Review of Respiratory Diseases,* **128,** 752-760.

West, J.B. (1984). Human physiology at extreme altitudes on Mount Everest. *Science,* **223,** 784-788.

Whipp, B. (1981). Control of exercise hyperpnea. In T.F. Hornbein (Ed.), *Regulation of breathing: Part II* (pp. 1069-1140). New York: Marcel Dekker.

Wilson, J.R., & Ferrara, N. (1983). Exercise intolerance in patients with chronic left heart failure: Relation to O_2 transport and ventilatory abnormalities. *American Journal of Cardiology,* **51,** 1358-1363.

Wright, J.L., Lawson, L., Paré, P.D., Hooper, R.O., Peretz, D.S., Nelems, J.M., Schulzer, M., & Hogg, J.C. (1983). The structure and function of the pulmonary vasculature in mild chronic obstructive pulmonary disease: The effects of oxygen and exercise. *American Review of Respiratory Disease,* **128,** 702-707.

The original studies reported in this paper were funded by NHLBI, USARDC, the H.M. Mayer Trust, and the University of Wisconsin Graduate School. We thank Ms. Pamela Hamm for her excellent preparation of the manuscript.

Chapter 11

Evaluation and Testing of the COPD Patient Prior to Rehabilitation

Gerilynn Connors

In 1981, the American Thoracic Society published an official position statement on pulmonary rehabilitation. This position statement defines pulmonary rehabilitation, the sequence of an appropriate treatment plan, components of a program, service required, and benefits and limitations of a program (Hodgkin et al., 1981). In 1974, a committee of the American College of Chest Physicians published the following definition of pulmonary rehabilitation:

> Pulmonary Rehabilitation may be defined as an art of medical practice wherein an individually tailored, multidisciplinary program is formulated which, through accurate diagnosis, therapy, emotional support and education, stabilizes or reverses both the physio- and psychopathology of pulmonary diseases and attempts to return the patient to the highest possible functional capacity allowed by his pulmonary handicap and overall life situation. (Petty, 1975)

The initial medical evaluation and diagnostic workup of a pulmonary rehabilitation candidate is important in making an accurate diagnosis, so an appropriate treatment plan can be implemented. In this chapter we will be discussing the evaluation and testing of the COPD patient in the following areas: history and physical examination, chest roentgenogram, electrocardiogram, pulmonary function tests, exercise, psychosocial factors, nutrition, activities of daily living, and education.

Chronic Obstructive Pulmonary Disease

The term *chronic obstructive pulmonary disease* (COPD) refers to asthma, chronic bronchitis, and emphysema, all being characterized by an increased resistance to airflow leading to varying degrees of shortness of breath, fatigue, wheezing, cough, or sputum production (see Figure 1). *Asthma* has been defined as intermittent attacks of airway obstruction lasting from a few months to many years (American Thoracic Society, 1962). Many categorize asthma into two basic types: extrinsic (immunologic or allergic) and intrinsic (nonimmunologic or nonallergic). *Chronic bronchitis* is defined as a daily cough, productive of sputum, for at least 3 months each year for 2 consecutive years (American Thoracic Society, 1962). *Emphysema* is defined as an enlargement of the distal air spaces with alveolar fragmentation and breakdown of the alveolar septa (Burton, 1984). Emphysema also leads to loss of lung elasticity. If the pathophysiology of COPD is understood, the physician is better able to outline a program that specifically meets the patient's needs.

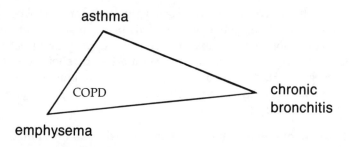

Figure 1 The term *chronic obstructive pulmonary disease* (COPD) refers to asthma, chronic bronchitis, and emphysema.

History and Physical Examination

The history and physical examination are important tools in the diagnosis of COPD (Hodgkin, 1979). The history should include the following: symptomatology, smoking history, drinking history, review of systems, medications taken, skin testing, and environmental health risk (Hodge-Hilton et al., 1984). Cough, sputum, shortness of breath, wheezing, edema, and chest pain are all symptoms that should be reviewed during the history.

The smoking history should include age of onset, number of tobacco products used each day, and type and pattern of smoking (inhaling, breath holding). The drinking history is important in determining its ef-

Table 1   Ingestion of Alcohol: Summary of Reported Problems Related to Lung Disease

---

Dehydrates cells
Alcohol metabolism unrelated to energy needs
Increases requirements for other nutrients
Decreases FVC
Decreases FEV_1
Decreases DL_{co}
Induces bronchoconstriction
Impairs clearance of bacteria from lungs
Impairs function of Type II alveolar cells
Alters $\dot{V}/Q$ matchup in lung
Increases metabolic acidosis
Interacts with adenylate cyclase
Enhances likelihood of sleep apnea

Note. From "Nutrition and the Pulmonary Patient" by J.A. Peters, K. Burke, and D. White, 1984, in J.E. Hodgkin, E.G. Zorn, and G.L. Connors (Eds.), *Pulmonary Rehabilitation: Guidelines to Success* (p. 271), Boston: Butterworth. Copyright 1984 by Butterworth Publishers. Reprinted by permission.

fect on behavior, activities of daily living, physical state, and compliance. Table 1 summarizes effects that alcohol has on COPD patients (Peters, Burke, & White, 1984). Review the systems for the presence of other diseases that the pulmonary rehabilitation client has and how they may relate to the patient's lung disease. Cardiac disease from right heart failure or cor pulmonale is often seen in patients with COPD. A hiatal hernia with esophageal reflux can lead to aspiration of stomach contents during sleep, leading to an exacerbation of asthma or chronic bronchitis. Postnasal drainage due to allergic rhinitis, vasomotor rhinitis, or chronic sinusitis can lead to aspiration of the secretions into the lungs at night and may also exacerbate asthma or cause bronchitis.

A review of past and current medications is important to determine proper dosages and potential side effects. If the patient is on digoxin or theophylline, checking a blood level can help optimum therapy. Theophylline is a methylxanthine drug which produces bronchodilation and has specific therapeutic responses related to the blood level of the drug (see Table 2). There are medications, e.g., propranolol, indomethicin, and aspirin, that may induce bronchoplasm in patients with asthma, so reviewing the patient's medication list is important.

Skin testing for specific allergens causing a patient's asthma may be helpful. Tuberculin skin testing may be useful in evaluating the patient with COPD.

Table 2 Therapeutic Responses Related to Blood Levels of Theophylline

Response	Blood Level of Theophylline
No effect	< 5 µg/ml
Suboptimal therapeutic level	5-9 µg/ml
Optimal therapeutic range	10-20 µg/ml
Anxiety may appear	> 15 µg/ml
GI toxicity likely	> 15 µg/ml
Usual toxic level	> 20 µg/ml
Arrhythmias likely to occur	> 30 µg/ml
Convulsions may occur	> 40 µg/ml

Note. From "Pharmacology and the Respiratory Patient" by A.R. Yee, G.L. Connor, and D.B. Cress, 1984, in J.E. Hodgkin, E.G. Zorn, and G.L. Connors (Eds.), *Pulmonary Rehabilitation: Guidelines to Success* (p. 129), Boston: Butterworth. Copyright 1984 by Butterworth Publishers. Reprinted by permission.

Exposure to on-the-job lung health hazards needs to be assessed, the length of exposure to any type of dust, fumes, or chemicals noted. The impact that pollution, both indoor and outdoor, has on the pulmonary patient may also be significant and should not be overlooked.

Once a thorough history is taken and the physical exam is completed, the physician orders appropriate diagnostic tests on the pulmonary rehabilitation client.

Chest Roentgenogram

The chest X ray can give an added perspective to the patient's cardiopulmonary status. The chest film may also be used to determine lung volumes accurately when obstructive airway disease is present (Burrows & Earle, 1969; Harris, Pratt, & Kilburn, 1971). Although the chest X ray is poor for the early diagnosis of COPD and in differentiating between asthma, chronic bronchitis, and emphysema, it is an important diagnostic tool. Findings to look for on a chest X ray include: sternodiaphragmatic angle greater than 90 degrees on a lateral view, a decrease in peripheral vascular markings, bullous changes, and flattened diaphragms, which are all common signs of emphysema. In chronic bronchitis, there may be an increase in the cardiovascular silhouette, suggesting pulmonary hypertension.

Electrocardiogram

The electrocardiogram is useful in detecting right ventricular hypertrophy, pulmonary hypertension, or evidence of ischemic heart disease. It should be monitored for arrhythmias and cardiac status, during exercise testing.

Pulmonary Function Tests

In this section the pulmonary function tests will be examined in regard to their application and assessment value relative to COPD.

Basic Spirometry

A pre- and post-bronchodilator spirogram is one of the least expensive of all the lung function tests. The forced vital capacity (FVC), forced expiratory volume in one second (FEV_1), and the forced expiratory flow over the mid 50% of the vital capacity (FEF 25-75%) are the parameters usually used to diagnose COPD (see Figure 2). The FEV_1 is felt by many to be the best predictor for prognosis and the most reliable for assessing the severity of lung function impairment (see Figure 3). The FEV_1/observed FVC is often reduced in early obstructive airway disease, even though the FEV_1 is normal, making this parameter more sensitive than the FEV_1 alone. The FEF 25-75% is a very sensitive test that can detect early obstructive airway disease (McFadden & Linden, 1972).

Maximum Voluntary Ventilation

The maximum voluntary ventilation (MVV) may be performed as part of basic spirometry. It is the volume of air the patient can breath in, fast and deep, during 12-15 seconds, expressed in l/min (see Figure 4). The results are very dependent upon patient endurance and cooperation.

An estimation of the MVV, by multiplying the FEV_1 by 35-40, has been reported to be a useful method for assessing the patient's ventilatory limits to exercise in conjunction with exercise testing (Clarke, Freedman, & Campbell, 1969; Freedman, 1970; Spiro, Holm, Edwards, & Pride, 1975).

Lung Volume Studies

Lung volume studies are determined by the helium dilution method, nitrogen washout technique, or with body plethysmography. Lung volume studies determine functional residual capacity (FRC), total lung

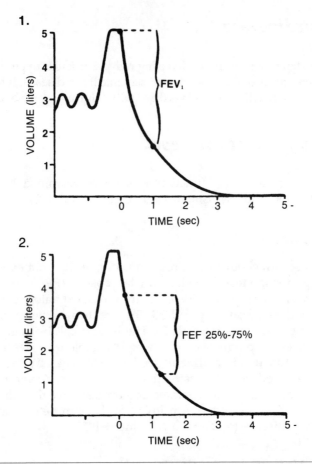

Figure 2 Spirometric tracings of (1) the forced expiratory volume in 1 second (FEV₁) and (2) the forced expiratory flow between 25% and 75% (FEF 25-75%) of the forced vital capacity.

capacity (TLC), and residual volume (RV) (see Figure 5). Total lung capacity can also be measured from a chest X ray (see roentgenogram section). The X-ray technique and body plethysmograph more reliably determine lung volumes than the gas dilution methods in patients with obstructive airway disease.

Diffusing Capacity

The diffusing capacity for carbon monoxide (DLco) measurement determines the ability of gases to diffuse across the alveolar-capillary membrane. It is a very sensitive indicator of early interstitial lung disease (i.e., pulmonary sarcoidosis) and may be reduced even when the TLC, arterial blood gas (ABG), and chest X ray are normal. The diagnosis of emphy-

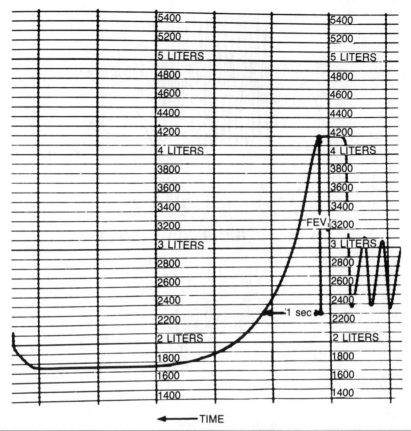

Figure 3 The forced expiratory volume in 1 second (FEV), is felt by many to be the best predictor for prognosis. *Note.* From *Respiratory Care: A Guide to Clinical Practice* (2nd ed., p. 233) by J.E. Hodgkin and G.G. Burton, 1984, Philadelphia: J.B. Lippincott. Copyright 1984 by J.B. Lippincott Company. Reprinted by permission.

sema can also be helped by measuring the DLco, which can be significantly reduced due to loss of alveolar-capillary membrane surface area.

Arterial Blood Gas Analysis

The monitoring of the arterial blood gas (ABG) is a basic part of the physiological evaluation of the pulmonary rehabilitation candidate. Determination of hypoxemia, ventilation-perfusion mismatch $(P(A-a)O_2)$, hypercapnia, and acid-base balance can be accomplished. A National Heart, Lung, and Blood Institute study done with hypoxemic COPD patients concluded that patients with a PaO_2 of 55mmHg or less and using supplemental oxygen only at nighttime had twice the mortality rate as those using oxygen continuously (Nocturnal Oxygen Therapy Trial Group, 1980). Through this study, guidelines have been developed for

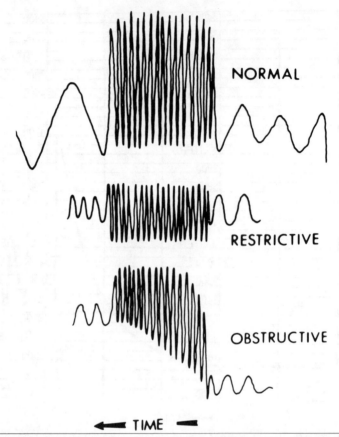

Figure 4 The maximum voluntary ventilation (MVV) is the volume of air the patient can breathe in, fast and deep, during 12-15 seconds, expressed in l/min. *Note.* From *Respiratory Care: A Guide to Clinical Practice* (2nd ed., p. 237) by J.E. Hodgkin and G.G. Burton, 1984, Philadelphia: J.B. Lippincott. Copyright 1984 by J.B. Lippincott Company. Reprinted by permission.

the administration of oxygen therapy. Analysis of the ABG (or oxygen saturation through ear oximetry) during exercise and sleep can provide useful information regarding the need for supplemental oxygen.

Pulmonary Exercise Stress Test

Exercise training in cardiac rehabilitation via aerobic exercise is widely accepted, but in rehabilitation of the COPD patient it has been questioned by some. There are many theories and ideas leading to the acceptance of exercise training in the COPD patient. The training response of bio-chemical and physiological-anatomic adaptations seen in the healthy and cardiovascular-diseased patient has been reported *not* to occur in the

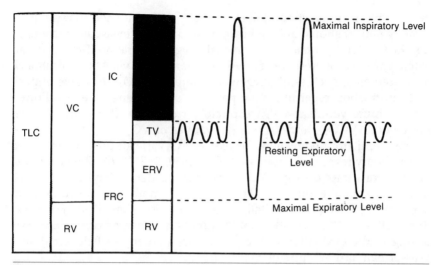

Figure 5   Lung value studies determine functional residual capacity (FRC), total lung capacity (TLC), and residual volume (RV). *Note.* From *The Lung: Clinical Physiology and Pulmonary Function Tests* (2nd ed., p. 8) by J.H. Comroe, Jr., R.E. Forster, II, A.B. DuBois, et al., 1962, Chicago: Year Book. Copyright 1962 by Year Book Medical Publishers. Reprinted by permission.

COPD patient (Belman & Kendregan, 1981). It is suggested that pulmonary patients may not be able to endure the level of exercise required for physiological-anatomic adaptations (Belman & Wasserman, 1981; Hughes & Davison, 1985).

To date there is no universally accepted and utilized pulmonary exercise stress test for evaluating and rehabilitating the pulmonary patient. The technology of metabolic and pulmonary measurements has been around for 10 years and is just now being accepted as a routine evaluation tool for pulmonary rehabilitation (Bell, Kass, & Hodgkin, 1983). The pulmonary stress tests used most in laboratories in the U.S. are a steady-state submaximal test and a progressive test to only submaximal levels, with few laboratories utilizing progressive tests that are continued to a symptom-limited or maximal level (Bell et al., 1983). These questions need to be answered:

- What data should one attempt to collect from the patient's exercise response?
- How can one best gather this data?
- How can this data be used to evaluate comprehensively the patient's physiologic status? (Bell et al., 1983)

The type of test Bell et al. (1983) have recommended to help answer these questions is the progressive test administered to a symptom-limited maximal level of exercise. The equipment available today to perform exercise stress testing is impressive, but consensus as to the variables to be collected is in question. Bell et al., have recommended that the pulmonary patient should at least be monitored for cardiovascular response, i.e., ECG, blood pressure, and arterial oxygen saturation (SaO_2) via ear oximetry or partial pressure of arterial oxygen (PaO_2) via ABG. Additional measurements, such as of oxygen consumption ($\dot{V}O_2$), can give important information regarding "the patient's specific energy expenditure, while minute ventilation $\dot{V}_E$, respiratory frequency (f), carbon dioxide production ($\dot{V}CO_2$), and various derivatives of $\dot{V}O_2$ and $\dot{V}CO_2$ (for example, ventilatory equivalent for oxygen [$O_2\dot{V}_E$]) can provide an index of ventilatory response to exercise" (Bell, 1980; Bell, 1976). The maximum oxygen consumption rate ($\dot{V}O_2$ max) can be determined from actual measurements of expired air. This provides a more accurate value than using prediction equations (Bell, Kass, Patil, & Repsher, 1980). For more information on the cardiorespiratory variables measured during exercise testing in the evaluation of the pulmonary patient see Bell (1980) and Wasserman and Whipp (1975).

Laboratory Tests

The following section outlines the most common laboratory tests used to assess COPD.

Sputum Analysis

In determining the presence of cells in purulent sputum, the Wright stain or wet mount technique for sputum analysis is widely used. Bronchial irritation with purulent sputum production can be due to an allergic process or an infection. Eosinophils predominate in an allergic problem, and steroid therapy may be indicated (Slim, Staver, & Williams, 1978); whereas neutrophils predominate in an infectious process, and antimicrobials would be the choice of treatment for a bacterial infection. The collection of a 24-hour sputum sample is helpful in order to quantitate both volume and consistency of production. Sputum collection for fungus, tuberculosis, and cytologic examination may be useful with certain patients. Sputum analysis for screening of malignant cells in patients at high risk of developing lung cancer is controversial, but it may occasionally detect lung cancer in an asymptomatic patient (Melamed, Flehinger, & Zaman, 1981; Taylor, Fontana & Uhlenhopp, 1981).

Complete Blood Count/Chemistry Profile

The complete blood count (CBC) and chemistry profile can give pertinent information regarding the patient's homeostasis or disease process. In the CBC the hemoglobin (Hgb), red blood cell count (RBC), hematocrit (Hct), mean cell hemoglobin concentration (MCHC), mean cell volume (MCV), and mean cell hemoglobin (MCH) can give information in regards to anemia or polycythemia, which can have significant impact on the COPD patient's oxygen status. The blood chemistry and electrolytes are important to monitor in a pulmonary patient because abnormalities in these constituents can affect the status of the patient's function.

Alpha₁ Antitrypsin Assay

A patient presenting with a family history of COPD, predominantly lower lobe emphysema (Mittman et al., 1972), early age onset of respiratory symptoms, or a documented family history of alpha₁ antitrypsin deficiency should get the alpha₁ antitrypsin assay. It is important to determine the persons at high risk and to direct education toward prevention and marital or genetic counseling when indicated (Mittman, Barbela, & Lieberman, 1973).

Polysomnography

Sleep-associated breathing disorders can have significant impact on the COPD patient. Pulmonary patients monitored during deep levels of sleep have shown a rise in arterial PCO_2 and a fall in PaO_2 (Koo, Sax, & Snider, 1975; Wynne, Block, & Hemerway, 1979), resulting in an increase in pulmonary artery pressure (Coccagna & Lugaresi, 1978). "Sleep studies should be performed in the face of pulmonary hypertension out of proportion to arterial hypoxemia, especially when symptoms or signs of sleep apnea syndrome are present" (Hodge-Hilton et al., 1984).

Psychosocial Evaluation and Testing

The psychosocial evaluation assesses the patient's current functional level and ego strength in order to help in developing a treatment plan. It allows an understanding of the patient's emotional states, educational abilities, support systems, and personal interest (Kaplan, 1979; Kim, Knecht, Hiscox, & Glaser, 1984; Kirscht, Becker, & Evalan, 1976; Prigatano, Wright, & Levin, 1984; Shontz & Fink, 1961).

There are a multitude of psychological tests that may be used in assessing the pulmonary patient. It is important that the tests used are simple enough so the administration, scoring or interpretation process is not complicated, but reliable and valid (Kim et al, 1984). Below is a list of the psychosocial tests that may be used on the pulmonary patient. The

Minnesota Multiphasic Personality Inventory (MMPI), and Wechsler and Rorschach tests will not be discussed here, even though they are well standardized, reliable, and valid, because they are very complicated.

Besle Index for Psychosocial Assets assesses the patient's social support system, coping ability, and adaptive ability. A patient rating 80% or greater has greater levels of compliance and performance.

Holmes and Rahe's Schedule of Recent Experience evaluates 43 life events to determine which life changes and stressors the patient is experiencing. The results show a relatively linear relationship between life changes and the probability of disease onset (Dudley & Sitzman, 1979).

OARS Social Resource Scale rates the patient's social relationships with significant others from "excellent social resources" to "total social impairment" (Kane & Kane, 1981).

Self-Rating Depression Scale (SDS) by Zung (1965) is composed of 20 items that are the common symptoms of a depressive disorder; through clinical correlation, the SDS can help evaluate a depressive patient.

Short Portable Mental Status Questionnaire (SPMQ) consists of 10 items and assesses organic brain deficiency in elderly patients. The results of evaluating the patient's intellectual functioning can assist in a clinical decision of self-care (Pfeiffer, 1975).

The Sickness Impact Profile (SIP) consists of 136 items in 12 areas of activity and focuses on the patient's perception of behavior and activity. It is designed to measure sickness-related behavioral dysfunction and is a valuable tool for assessing the patient's health-related behavioral performance and the outcome of a rehabilitation program (Pollard, Bobbitt, Bergner, Martin, & Gilson, 1976).

The precise role that psychological testing should play in evaluating the pulmonary rehabilitation client is yet to be determined.

Nutritional Evaluation/Testing

Food and air are essential for life, but the nutritional status of the COPD outpatient is often overlooked. The emphysemic "pink puffer" patient is often underweight, whereas the chronic bronchitic "blue bloater" is often normal or overweight (Peters, Burke, & White, 1984). There are a variety of reasons for the poor nutritional status of many pulmonary patients. Some of these reasons are (a) a feeling of fullness, (b) abdominal distention, (c) shortness of breath, (d) diminished sense of smell, (e) medications, and (f) peptic ulcers. The result can be protein-energy malnutrition, causing immunoincompetence and increased susceptibility to respiratory infections.

The diet commonly recommended for the pulmonary patient is high complex carbohydrate (CHO) and low fat. Carbohydrate has been reported to increase levels of 2,3 DPG, thereby increasing tissue oxygenation (Blankenship et al., 1977). A high-fat-content diet can induce angina pectoris in cardiac patients by increasing blood lipid levels that affect oxygenation (Kao & Joyner, 1955). High fat intake also causes a reduction in the intake of CHO and "is associated with an elevated risk of heart disease, breast and colon cancer" (Select Committee on Nutrition and Human Needs, 1977). Starvation has also been found to cause emphysema-like changes in the lung (Keys, Brozek, Henschel, Mickelson, & Taylor, 1950), so this is another important reason for proper nutrition in the pulmonary patient.

During the physical examination, attention should be given to the patient's hair changes, skin changes, mental confusion, hepatomegaly, pitting edema, ascites, or a scaphoid abdomen (Peters et al., 1984).

Anthropometric Methods

The patient's height and weight should be measured. Triceps skinfold thickness should be assessed, because it is a good estimate of subcutaneous fat; a low thickness may indicate protein-energy deprivation, whereas a high thickness indicates chronic overconsumption of calories. Skeletal muscle mass and arm fat area are other simple, non-invasive measurements that can help to determine skeletal muscle mass (Peters et al., 1984).

Laboratory Tests

There are a multitude of laboratory tests that can be done to assess the patient's state of nutrition. These are not routine screening tests, but may be indicated after a complete history and physical examination. The creatinine-height index can provide an estimate of protein-energy malnutrition by estimating the amount of total skeletal muscle mass. Serum albumin is the most important component in the bloodstream for determining collidal oncotic pressure in order to help prevent edema; the test correlates well with body protein reserves of muscle mass. Serum transferrin binds and transports iron, and the blood test reflects early changes in protein-energy nutrition. "Nitrogen balance, if negative, may indicate inadequate absorption of protein quality, quantity, too little energy, or any combination of these" (Peters et al., 1984). Prealbumin and retinol-binding proteins are sensitive parameters to estimate protein-energy nutrition.

Activities of Daily Living Evaluation/Testing

The COPD patient, due to dyspnea and fatigue, often experiences a decrease in the ability to perform activities of daily living (see Figure 6). It is important for the patient to maintain his role and function in society. Evaluation of upper extremity range of motion, strength, coordination, sensation, and function needs to be accomplished (Shanfield & Hammond, 1984). Common problems seen in the COPD patient include (Shanfield & Hammond, 1984):

- decreased range of motion in the shoulders,
- tremors and incoordination,
- decreased sensation in the forearm or hands,
- decreased endurance.

Physiological monitoring with ECG telemetry during activities is the most accurate way to determine safe activity guidelines for the patient. Monitoring heart rate, blood pressure, and symptomatic responses to the activity are also important. Portable ear oximetry is useful in assessing a patient's oxygen level during activity.

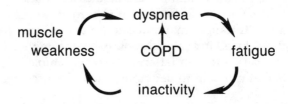

Figure 6 The COPD inactivity cycle is self-perpetuating and difficult to break.

Educational Evaluation/Testing

Pre-evaluation and testing to diagnose a disease is widely accepted; however, when one begins to speak of an educational diagnosis, there is often silence. Although "the state of the art in education at this time does not provide definite tests to employ in making an educational diagnosis" (Hopp & Maddox, 1984, p. 52), there are a few tools that may be helpful.

The Health Belief Model

The Health Belief Model is a predictor of the likelihood of a patient to take preventive or therapeutic action, based on five perceptual areas or beliefs: (a) seriousness or severity of the disease, (b) the patient's susceptibility, (c) threatened damage from the disease, (d) benefits of action and (e) barriers to taking action (Becker, 1974; Hopp & Maddox, 1984). To test and assess a patient's beliefs about a given disease, one does not need a written test, but one does need to *listen* to the patient.

Multidimensional Health Locus of Control

The Multidimensional Health Locus of Control is a simple two-page questionnaire derived from Rotter's social learning theory, developed by Wallston, Wallston, and DeVellis (1978). It shows the patient's view of the world and perception about his degree of control over events that happen to him. "If the person perceives that an event is contingent upon luck, fate, or chance, or upon powerful others, the person is said to have an external locus of control (Hopp & Maddox, 1984, pp. 48-49). This person believes he has no control over events. The persons who believe that "events are contingent upon their own decisions or behaviors are internal individuals" (Hopp & Maddox, p. 49). Again, just through listening to patients, one may determine if the patient is internal or external. Most patients are never purely internal or external, but tend more toward one end of the scale or the other. It is important that the educational program meet the needs of each pulmonary patient.

Summary

There are numerous tests and evaluations that can be done on pulmonary rehabilitation candidates. The ATS statement on pulmonary rehabilitation stresses the importance of diagnostic workup and evaluation. The following is a list of the basic medical tests that should be considered for every pulmonary rehabilitation candidate:

- Chest X ray, PA and lateral
- CBC
- Blood chemistry profile
- ECG
- Prepost bronchodilator spirometry test
- DLco
- Total lung capacity
- Pulmonary exercise stress test
- Room air ABG
- Blood theophylline level (if the patient is taking a theophylline medication)
- Sputum examination

The evaluation and testing of the psychosocial, ADL, nutritional, and educational components of the patient's current status should also be assessed.

Through a careful assessment of the pulmonary rehabilitation candidate, a program that meets the patient's needs can be developed. That's what pulmonary rehabilitation is all about!

References

American Thoracic Society (Committee on Diagnostic Standards for Non-Turberculous Respiratory Diseases). (1962). Definitions and classification of chronic bronchitis, asthma, and pulmonary emphysema. *American Review of Respiratory Disease, 85,* 762-768.

Becker, M.H. (1974). *The health belief model and personal health behavior.* Thorofare, NJ: Slack.

Bell, C.W. (1976). Exercise stress testing and physical conditioning program. In I. Kass (Ed.), *Pulmonary rehabilitation medical manual* (pp. 50-91). Omaha: University of Nebraska Press.

Bell, C.W. (1980). Pulmonary rehabilitation and exercise testing. In P.K. Wilson, C.W. Bell, & A.C. Norton (Eds.), *Rehabilitation of the heart and lungs* (p. 54). Fullerton, CA: Beckman Instruments.

Bell, C.W., Kass, I., & Hodgkin, J.E. (1983). Exercise conditioning. In J.F. Hodgkin, E.G. Zorn, & G.L. Connors (Eds.), *Pulmonary rehabilitation: Guidelines to success* (pp.195-206). Boston: Butterworths.

Bell, C.W., Kass, I., Patil, K.D., & Repsher, L.H. (1980). Relationship of pulmonary function variables and maximal oxygen consumption rate in the determination of disability in patients with chronic obstructive pulmonary disease (abstract). *American Review of Respiratory Disease, 121,* 223.

Belman, M.J., & Kendregan, B.A. (1981). Exercise training fails to increase skeletal muscle enzymes in patients with chronic obstructive pulmonary disease. *American Reveiw of Respiratory Disease, 123,* 256-261.

Belman, M.J., & Wasserman, K. (1981). Exercise training and testing in patients with chronic obstructive pulmonary disease. *Basics of RD,* (Pub, ATS-ALA, NY) 10:1-6.

Blankenship, J.W., Dassenko, S., Johnson, L., Register, U.D., Vyhmeister, I.B., & Yahiku, P.Y. (1977). Effect of diet on serum cholesterol and triglyceride levels and red blood cell 2, 3-diphosphoglycerate level. *Federation Proceedings, 36,* 1104.

Burrows, B., & Earle, R.H. (1969). Course and prognosis of chronic obstructive lung disease: A prospective study of 200 patients. *New England Journal of Medicine, 280,* 397-404.

Burton, G.G. (1984). Differential diagnosis of the various obstructive pulmonary diseases and implications for therapy. In G.G. Burton & J.E. Hodgkin (Eds.), *Respiratory care: A guide to clinical practice* (2nd ed.). Philadelphia: Lippincott.

Clark, T.J.H., Freedman, S., & Campbell, E.J.M. (1969). The ventilatory capacity of patients with chronic airway obstruction. *Clinical Science,* **36**, 307-316.

Coccagna, G., & Lugaresi, E. (1978). Arterial blood gases and pulmonary and systematic arterial pressure during sleep in chronic obstructive pulmonary disease. *Sleep,* **1**, 117-124.

Dudley, D.L., & Sitzman, J. (1979). Psychosocial and psychophysiologic approach to the patient. *Seminars in Respiratory Medicine,* **1**, 59-82.

Freedman, S. (1970). Sustained maximum voluntary ventilation. *Respiratory Physiology,* **8**, 230-244.

Harris, T.R., Pratt, P.C., & Kilburn, K.H. (1971). Total lung capacity measured by roentgenograms. *American Journal of Medicine,* **50**, 756-763.

Hodge-Hilton, T., Herrmann, D.W., et al. (1984). Initial evaluation of the pulmonary rehabilitation candidate. In J.F. Hodgkin, E.G. Zorn, & G.L. Connors (Eds.), *Pulmonary rehabilitation: Guidelines to success.* Boston: Butterworths.

Hodgkin, J.E. (1979). *Chronic obstructive pulmonary disease: Current concepts in diagnosis and comprehensive care.* Chicago: ACCP.

Hodgkin, J.E., Farrell, M.J., Gibson, S.R., et al. (1981). Pulmonary rehabilitation: Official ATS statement. *American Review of Respiratory Disease,* **124**, 663-666.

Hopp, J.W., & Maddox, S.E. (1984). Education of patients and their families. In J.E. Hodgkin, E.G. Zorn, & G.L. Connors (Eds.), *Pulmonary rehabilitation: Guidelines to success* (pp. 45-62). Boston: Butterworths.

Hughes, R.L., & Davison, R. (1983). Limitations of exercise reconditioning in COLD. *Chest,* **83**, 241-249.

Kane, R., & Kane, R. (1981). *Assessing the elderly: A practical guide to measurement.* Lexington, MA: D.C. Health.

Kao, P.T., & Joyner, C.R. (1955). Angina pectoris induced by fat ingestion in patients with coronary artery disease. *Journal of the American Medical Association,* **158**(12), 1008-1013.

Kaplan, H.B. (1979). Social psychology of disease. In H. Freeman, S. Levine, & L.G. Reeder (Eds.), *Handbook of medical sociology* (pp. 53-96). Englewood Cliffs, NJ: Prentice-Hall.

Keys, A.J., Brozek, A., Henschel, A., Mickelsen, D., & Taylor, H.L. (1950). *The biology of human starvation.* Minneapolis: University of Minnesota Press.

Kim, H.T., Knecht, P.A., Hiscox, D.E., & Glaser, E.M. (1984). Psychosocial factors and pulmonary patients. In J.E. Hodgkin, E.G. Zorn,

& G.L. Connors (Eds.), *Pulmonary rehabilitation: Guidelines to success* (pp. 207-238). Boston: Butterworths.

Kirsht, J.P., Becker, M.H., & Evelan, J.P. (1976). Psychological and social factors as predictors of medical behavior. *Medical Care, 14*, 422-431.

Koo, K.W., Sax, D.S., & Snider, G.L. (1975). Arterial blood gas and pH during sleep in chronic obstructive pulmonary disease. *American Journal of Medicine, 48*, 663-670.

McFadden, E.R., Jr., & Linden, D.A. (1972). A reduction in maximum midexpiratory flow rate: A spirographic manifestation of small airway disease. *American Journal of Medicine, 52*, 725.

Melamed, M.R., Flehinger, B.J., & Zaman, M.B. (1981). Detection of true pathological stage, lung cancer in a screening program and the effect on survival. *Cancer, 47*, 1182-1187.

Miller, R.D., & Offord, K.P. (1980). Roentgenologic determination of total lung capacity. *Mayo Clinic Proceedings, 55*, 694-699.

Mittman, C., Barbela, T., & Lieberman, J. (1973). Alpha$_1$ antitrypsin deficiency as an indicator of susceptibility of pulmonary disease. *Journal of Occupational Medicine, 15*, 33-38.

Mittman, C., Lieberman, J., Marasso, F., et al. (1972). Summary of symposium on pulmonary emphysema and proteolysis. *American Review of Respiratory Disease, 105*, 430-448.

Nocturnal Oxygen Therapy Trial Group. (1980). Continuous vs. nocturnal oxygen therapy in hypoxemic chronic obstructive lung disease. *Annals of Internal Medicine, 93*, 391-398.

Peters, J.A., Burke, K., & White, D. (1984). Nutrition and the pulmonary patient. In J.E. Hodgkin, E.G. Zorn, & G.L. Connors (Eds.), *Pulmonary rehabilitation: Guidelines to success* (pp. 263-298). Boston: Butterworth.

Petty, T.L. (1975). Pulmonary rehabilitation. *Basics of RD*, New York: American Thoracic Society.

Pfeiffer, E. (1975). A short, portable mental status questionnaire for the assessment of organic brain deficit in elderly patients. *American Geriatrics Society, 23*(10), 433-441.

Pollard, W.E., Bobbitt, R.A., Bergner, M., Martin, D.P., & Gilson, B.S. (1976). The sickness impact profile: Reliability of a health status measure. *Medical Care, 14*(2), 146-155.

Prigatano, G.P., Wright, E.C., & Levin, D. (1984). Quality of life and its predictors in patients with mild hypoxemia and chronic obstructive pulmonary disease. *Archives of Internal Medicine, 144*, 1613-1619.

Select Committee on Nutrition and Human Needs, United States Senate. (1977). *Diet and killer diseases with press reaction and additional information*. Washington, DC: U.S. Government Printing Office.

Shanfield, K., & Hammond, M.A. (1984). Activities of daily living. In J.E. Hodgkin, E.G. Zorn, & G.L. Connors (Eds.), *Pulmonary rehabilitation: Guidelines to success* (pp. 171-193). Boston: Butterworths.

Shontz, F.C., & Fink, S.L. (1961). A method for evaluating psychosocial adjustments of chronically ill. *American Journal of Physical Medicine,* **40**(2), 63-69.

Slim, C., Staver, D.E., & Williams, M.H., Jr. (1978). Response to corticosteroids in chronic bronchitis. *Journal of Allergy and Clinical Immunology,* **62**, 363-367.

Spiro, S.G., Holm, H.L., Edwards, R.H.T., & Pride, N.B. (1975). An analysis of the physiologic strain of submaximal exercise in patients with chronic obstructive bronchitis. *Thorax,* **30**, 415-425.

Taylor, W.F., Fontana, R.S., & Uhlenhopp, M.A. (1981). Some results of screening for early lung cancer. *Cancer,* **47**, 1114-1120.

Wallston, K.A., Wallston, B.S., & DeVellis, R. (1978). Development of the multidimensional health locus of control (MHLC) scales. *Health Education Monographs,* **46**(2), 160-170.

Wasserman, K., & Whipp, B.J. (1975). Exercise physiology in health and disease. *American Reveiw of Respiratory Disease,* **112**, 219-249.

Wynne, J.W., Block, A.J., & Hemerway, J. (1979). Disordered breathing and oxygen desaturation in patients with chronic obstructive lung disease (COLD). *American Journal of Medicine,* **66**, 573-579.

Zung, W.W.K. (1965). A self-rating depression scale. *Archives of General Psychiatry,* **12**, 63-70.

I would like to express my gratitude to John E. Hodgkin, M.D., who took time from his busy schedule to edit the chapter.

Chapter 12

COPD: Exercise, Psychological Support, and Education

Catherine Reith Murphy

Chronic obstructive pulmonary disease (COPD), which includes chronic bronchitis, emphysema, and asthma, differs from other devastating illness in its lack of a critical incident. The disability is insidious, yet invisible, and patients usually seek medical attention only when their disease is advanced. By this time symptoms are burdensome, and the disability is rapidly overtaking the life and happiness of the patient. For these reasons, COPD remains a significant challenge to the medical community. However, approaches to rehabilitate individuals with disabling dyspnea have emerged (Butts, 1981; Petty & Nelt, 1978).

At its annual meeting in 1974, the American College of Chest Physicians' Committee on Pulmonary Rehabilitation adopted the following definition:

> Pulmonary rehabilitation may be defined as an art of medical practice wherein an individually tailored, multidisciplinary program is formulated that, through accurate diagnosis, therapy, emotional support, and education, stabilizes or reverses both the physio- and the psychopathy of pulmonary diseases and attempts to return the patient to the highest possible functional capacity allowed by his pulmonary handicap and overall life situation. (Petty & Nelt, 1978, p. 28)

Pulmonary rehabilitation should focus on maximizing the patient's improvement and minimizing the impact of the illness. To achieve these goals optimally, the rehabilitation program must be directed toward the patient and family, and include exercise, education and psychological support.

Exercise

Exercise plays an integral role in the rehabilitation of patients with COPD. It serves to break the vicious cycle of deconditioning that is so much a part of the disease. The chronic dyspnea, or shortness of breath, leads to fear and anxiety about physical activity. Further deconditioning continues as a more sedentary lifestyle is undertaken to prevent the symptoms. Exercise rehabilitation concurrent with education provides COPD patients with an alternative and, if initiated early in the disease process, may slow the degenerative effects of COPD (Bell, 1980; Shephard, 1976).

Prior to beginning an exercise program, the COPD patient should be given a thorough assessment, including structural, functional, and orthopedic evaluations. Exercise tests should be designed to identify any cardiopulmonary limitations to exercise, as well as the patient's physical work capacity. Tests should also be designed to yield specific, practical information that will help in planning the training program (Butts, 1981). The results of the exercise test and initial evaluation provide the necessary information for writing the exercise prescription.

Exercise Prescription

An exercise program should consist of a warm-up, stimulus period, and cool-down. The warm-up and cool-down include low-intensity aerobic activity and stretching. The stimulus period must provide four essential components that are the foundation of the exercise prescription: intensity, duration, frequency, and mode.

Intensity: Intensity is usually prescribed by taking a straight percentage of a person's maximal functional capacity. The American College of Sports Medicine (1980) suggests that intensities ranging between 60-90% of maximum heart rate or 50-85% of the maximal volume of oxygen consumed ($\dot{V}O_2$ max) are needed to induce positive training effects.

However, in a pulmonary population this creates quite a challenge, for patients with respiratory disease are limited because of their dyspnea before achieving a true maximal value. Therefore, alternative methods must be explored. One such method is to determine a straight percentage of the patient's "maximal tolerable heart rate" (HR_T max) (Bell, 1980). The heart rate range should be between 60-85% of the HR_T max. Some persons may not be able to tolerate such a heart rate initially; it may be necessary to adjust the prescription heart rate downward and then progressively increase it (over days or weeks) as their exercise tolerance improves (Bell, 1980).

Another option for assessing intensity is the measurement of anaerobic threshold. The anaerobic threshold is a point in the exercise when there is a greater demand for oxygen than there is supply. If exercise is prescribed too far below the anaerobic threshold, the patient probably will not derive the fitness adaptation sought through training. On the other hand, if the intensity is set above the anaerobic threshold, the training sessions may be unsafe and discourage compliance because of the vigor of the workout. Therefore, it is useful to measure the anaerobic threshold during the exercise test and key the prescription slightly below its onset. Measurement of the anaerobic threshold can be obtained noninvasively by examining the slope of the curve of V_E plotted against work. If $\dot{V}O_2$ and $\dot{V}CO_2$ are being measured, an even closer estimate of this point can be made (Bell, 1980).

In some COPD patients, assigning a specific pulse rate or heart rate range may be inappropriate because of their severe physical limitations (Brown, Fregosi, & Reddan, 1982). For these persons duration should be the primary focus, with attempts to attain a 20-30% increase above the resting heart rate (Frownfelter, 1979a).

Duration: In order to obtain a training effect, 15-60 minutes of aerobic activity is required (American College of Sports Medicine, 1980). Of course, the COPD patient cannot be expected to work for that amount of time at the onset of the program. He will need to proceed at his own pace and gradually increase his exercise time increments.

Frequency: The frequency of the conditioning program ultimately determines its success. The COPD patient just starting will be doing exercise of less duration per session and, therefore, should be instructed to exercise more often. Two to three short (3-5 minutes) periods of exercise each day would not be inappropriate (O'Ryan, 1984b). Ideally the COPD patient should exercise at least 3 to 5 times per week.

Mode: Cardiopulmonary fitness is best achieved through any activity that uses large muscle groups, can be maintained continuously, and is rhythmical and aerobic in nature. Realistic modes of exercise for COPD patients consist of walking, cycling, or stair climbing. The modes can be performed separately each session, resulting in continuous training, or combined for more of a circuit-interval approach. Whenever possible, exercise should be task-specific (i.e., walking to the store, newspaper stand, etc.) (O'Ryan, 1984).

Because of the specificity of training, a COPD exercise program should involve training of muscles that are used in activities the patient considers most important. In a study by Paez, Phillipson, and Massongkay (1967), emphysema patients who used a bicycle ergometer, and then a treadmill, were tested for the degree of training effect present when they used the bicycle a second time. Only a minimal effect was transferred from the treadmill to the bicycle. The results support the concept of training specificity.

With this concept in mind, one must not overlook arm training. Arm muscles can become just as deconditioned from prolonged disuse as leg muscles. Use of arm muscle groups is required for normal activities of daily living and benefits of leg training are not transferable. Arm work is usually performed extremely inefficiently and results in dyspnea and fatigue. Many patients hold their breath until an arm task is completed and must recover not only from the stress of performing the task with weakened arms, but also from breathing irregularity. Because of these functional limitations, arm cycling and gravity-resisted arm exercises should be included in the training program.

Arm cycling is usually begun by pedaling against resistance for as long as the patient can tolerate. Gravity-resisted arm exercises (i.e., arm circles and arm raises) should be performed at gradually increasing intervals and repetitions. Combined with the lower leg training program, arm training can further increase tolerance for daily living, recreational, and vocational activities.

Supplemental Oxygen Requirements

In COPD patients, exercise-induced hypoxia is a possible problem. Patients who are not on oxygen may require supplemental oxygen while exercising. Patients already on oxygen may need to increase the flow. As early as 1956, evidence showed that use of supplemental oxygen is beneficial in improving exercise tolerance (Cotes & Gilson). Later, Vyas, Banister, and Morton (1971) showed that when COPD patients exercise with 40% oxygen, the oxygen equivalent is lower than when they exercise without it. Therefore, less ventilation is required to deliver each liter of oxygen.

Evidence for use of supplemental oxygen during exercise should be both subjective and objective. Oxygen is typically prescribed during exercise when ear oximetry shows that arterial desaturation is less than 85%. During the exercise tolerance test, the oxygen flow level should be recorded and used in the exercise prescription. Supplemental oxygen is usually supplied by nasal prongs at 1-4 L/min, or through a large, oxygen-enriched air reservoir that allows control of oxygen concentration.

Benefits of Exercise

In 1952, Barach was the first to encourage ambulation and activity of COPD patients, having noticed that active patients appeared to function better than their inactive counterparts. Since that time, many studies on the effects of exercise for COPD patients have been done, using a variety of exercise modes, durations, intensities, frequencies, and various types of patients. A wide variety of findings has been recorded, but consistently—regardless of exercise mode or patient type—an increased ability to exercise with decreased oxygen consumption has been documented (Miller, Taylor, & Pierce, 1963; Paez et al., 1967; Woolf & Swero, 1969). Interestingly, studies reveal that there is little change in pulmonary function, exercise heart rate, or cellular characteristics after training, in spite of increases in endurance capacity (Belman & Wasserman, 1982). Several mechanisms have been suggested by Belman and Wasserman for the increase in exercise capacity without change in lung function seen in pulmonary patients: (a) increased peripheral oxygen use, due to increased peripheral blood flow; (b) increased motivation; (c) desensitization to the sensation of dyspnea; (d) improved muscle function; and (e) improved technique of performance.

While exercise programs can be prescribed by utilizing specific testing measures, and their benefits can often be demonstrated by measurable results, the impact of psychological support is less quantifiable. This, of course, does not mean its role in a patient's life is less important. In the following section, I will discuss psychological support and the COPD patient.

Psychological Support

Dudley (1980) emphasizes that the COPD patient lives in a constant state of stress and suggests that his life is an "emotional straight jacket" (p. 413). The COPD patient cannot become angry, depressed, or happy, or experience any other emotional change, without risking shortness of breath. Furthermore, COPD patients tend to be extremely nervous and tense, often not knowing whether their next breath will even come (Holliday, 1984). Anxiety and depression are the most frequently encountered, and perhaps the most disabling, emotions accompanying COPD (Dudley et al., 1980).

Because anxiety and tension are strong factors in producing shortness of breath, psychological support is an essential component of the pulmonary rehabilitation process. Stress, anxiety, and depression can worsen existing physical and psychological problems and even weaken the body's ability to fight disease. The first step in providing psychological support is to identify the problem. Identification includes both subjective and objective assessments of the patient. Common anxiety symptoms are described in Table 1 (Blodgett, 1982).

A psychological assessment scale that can be administered to determine depression is the Beck Depression Inventory (Beck, 1972). This inventory assesses an individual's mood, self-concept, and somatic functioning, in order to determine the level of depression at the time of test administration. The Zung Depression Inventory (1965) also can be used to assess depression; however, it has been used primarily in the geriatric population. In addition to depression scales, the State-Trait Anxiety Inventory

Table 1 Common Anxiety Symptoms

Affective (Emotional) Symptoms	Cognitive (Mental) Symptoms	Physiological Symptoms	Psychomotor Symptoms
Irritability	Inability to concentrate	Headaches	Restlessness
Frequent mood changes	Short attention span	Muscle aches	Rapid or nervous speech pattern
Frequent feelings of guilt	Low efficiency	Frequent fatigue	Fidgeting
		Heavy perspiration	Overeating
		Dry mouth	Muscle tremors, tics
		Shortness of breath	
		Stomach disorders (e.g., indigestion, diarrhea, butterflies)	
		Increased heart rate and palpitations	
		Insomnia	

Note. From ''Relaxation Techniques'' by D. Blodgett, 1984, in C.W. Bell et al. (Eds.), *Home Care and Rehabilitation in Respiratory Medicine*, Philadelphia: J.B. Lippincott. Copyright 1982 by J.B. Lippincott Company. Reprinted by permission.

can be implemented to assess anxiety (Spielberg, 1968). An extremely helpful assessment tool is the Sickness Impact Profile (S.I.P.). This profile assesses the patient's perception of his health status relative to his performance of various activities of daily living. The Semantic Differential Scale (Meissner, 1980) assesses the patient's self-concept, which will affect how well he assimilates information. This tool can also provide feedback as to whether the content taught is having a positive effect on the patient's self-concept and is helping him regain control of his life.

Identification of psychological stress and its relationship to shortness of breath is important. Many patients report that when it is made clear that psychological stress increases, but does not directly cause, shortness of breath, they become aware from their own observations that shortness of breath can be triggered by stress (Holliday, 1984). Awareness of this association is critical in order for intervention to be effective.

Various techniques can be incorporated into the rehabilitation process to control pyschological stress. The major intervention thrust is to elicit a state of relaxation. Relaxation techniques can decrease stress, heart rate, and oxygen consumption. They can also slow respiratory rates and relieve anxiety. The goals of teaching relaxation techniques are to provide the patient with the feeling of control over anxiety, stress, and tension, and to allow him or her to participate in activities without being fearful (Blodgett, 1982). The most common techniques for relaxation include Benson's relaxation response, Jacobsen's progressive relaxation, yoga, meditation, and hypnosis (Frownfelter, 1979).

Biofeedback is a more recent relaxation technique. Biofeedback is essentially a process by which information about some physiological function that it is important for the patient to control is fed back to him through instrumentation (Holliday, 1984). Information is immediately given to the patient concerning his or her biologic functions, such as muscle tension, heart rate, and skin surface temperature. Holliday and Munz (1978) have suggested that biofeedback induces benefits beyond simple relaxation. Biofeedback gives the person a sense of control of his own body, or at least a belief that he could become able to control it. Of course, this ability would be very important in pulmonary rehabilitation, particulary in the management of dyspnea (Holliday, 1984). Holliday suggests that health professionals seeking certification in biofeedback should write to the address below for information:

Biofeedback Certification Institute of America
4301 Owens street
Wheat Ridge, CO 80033
(303) 420-2902

Regardless of the relaxation technique that is used, a quiet, reassuring therapist is often the best choice for teaching the procedure. The psychological benefits of exercise and education—not only those of relaxation techniques—should not be overlooked. The emotional benefits of exercise have been compiled by Ledwidge (1980). With continued, aerobic activity there are three essential benefits.

- Increase in self-esteem: This leads to increased confidence, which is usually generated by an improvement in the patient's body and a sense of accomplishment in overcoming physical challenges.
- Decrease in anxiety: The muscle action potential is typically increased in anxious and depressed patients. Exercise is known to reduce this. Research on the biochemistry of anxiety shows that lactate plays a key role in producing anxiety symptoms. Lactate is created by the chronic overproduction of adrenalin; aerobic training is known to reduce the amount of lactate. Finally, exercise promotes sound sleep. In fact, Ledwidge (1980) has surmised that exercise is the only behavioral manipulation proven to increase amounts of slow-wave sleep.
- Decrease in depression: Norepinephrine is notably low in depressed patients and exercise dramatically increases it. Also, chronic fatigue, a common complaint in depression, is relieved through exercise (Ledwidge, 1980).

It is believed that psychological interventions that are a routine part of patient and family education and therapy become gradually less obtrusive and thereby more acceptable. Furthermore, in a report of a 15-month patient education study prepared for the American Lung Association, Seiler (1979) indicated that education programs elicit positive, and apparently significant and long-lasting, changes in the COPD patient's psychological well-being.

Self-help and mutual support groups are also helpful in the psychological support of the pulmonary rehabilitation candidate. Organizations in an increasing number of states are collecting and disseminating information about local self-help groups and resources. These efforts are coordinated by the National Self-Help Clearing House (Graduate School and University Center/CUNY, 33 W. 42 St., New York, NY 10026) (Plummer, 1984). Gartner and Riessman, codirectors of the National Self-Help Clearing House, feel that self-help groups "provide social support to their members through the creation of a caring community, and they increase members' coping skills through the provision of information and the sharing of experiences and solutions to problems" (1982). Facilitation of the rehabilitation process is thus based upon a philosophy of the patient being a whole person not just a pair of lungs. Intervention should be designed to assist the patient in reformulating his or her self-concept based on worth, rather than on being a defective or deficient person (Plummer, 1984).

Education is another key aspect of any comprehensive pulmonary rehabilitation program. In the last section of this article, I will explore education topics that are important to COPD patients, and present educational resources that are currently available.

Education

Patient education is an essential component of any pulmonary rehabilitation program. To be most effective, it should involve the spouse and other family members. Patients must understand in simple terms lung structure and function, the disease process, its pathogenesis, symptoms of exacerbations, and the goals and specifics of therapy. The informed patient must become involved in his own care. Personalized and detailed instructions should be taught by someone—often a nurse, therapist, or technician—who has the requisite training, sufficient time, and patience to present the complex and sometimes difficult material to patients with a variety of educational backgrounds (Petty & Nelt, 1978). The educational process incorporates several disciplines and is often met through a team approach. Team members may include the physician, nurse coordinator, physical and occupational therapists, vocational counselor, recreation therapist, dietitian, respiratory therapist, pharmacist, and social worker.

The way that the patient feels about himself and the disease affects compliance with prescribed therapy. Perceptions of the diagnosis and severity of the disease, belief in the effectiveness of the program, and the lack of foreseeable obstacles affect the degree of compliance (Butts, 1981). To be successful, education must be comprehensive in scope, but individualized to meet specific patient and family needs.

Educational Topics

Frownfelter (1979) suggested that the following topics and content be included to complete the education component of the pulmonary rehabilitation process:

Respiratory Anatomy and Physiology: There should be a general discussion of the ciliary clearance mechanism and the cough. Audiovisual aids can be used to demonstrate the tracheobronchial tree segments and the different angles at which they take off from the main-stem bronchus. This assists in explaining postural drainage. Oxygen transport and the interdependency of the heart and lungs should also be discussed.

Environmental Irritation: This may be external or personal. Subjects such as paint fumes, smoking, extremes in environmental conditions, altitudes, and air travel should be discussed.

Infection: A patient should take preventive injections (influenza shots) at the physician's discretion. The patient should avoid friends with colds and should not become overly run-down.

Fluid Intake: A respiratory patient should be encouraged to increase fluid intake to 10-12 glasses (2 1/3-3 quarts) per day, unless there are cardiac problems because of which fluid intake should be restricted. Generally, fluids should not be extremely hot or cold because extremes can cause airway irritation. Ankle edema and sudden weight gain should be reported to the physician.

Nutrition: A dietitian is instrumental to the rehabilitation team for providing sound nutritional guidelines. Many respiratory patients lose their appetites and weight; anorexia is common. Often patients who are dyspneic swallow air; this, combined with irritating medications, can lead to nausea. Several small meals a day may provide better nutrition than the usual three big ones. Supplemental vitamins should be considered.

Medications: A patient needs to know what medications he or she is taking, and about their potential synergistic effects and side effects. Symptoms to watch for are mainly related to bronchodilators and include heart palpitations, tremors, insomnia, nausea, vomiting, urinary retention, anorexia, irritability, and personality changes. Extremes in symptoms are probably related to a toxic level of medication. Teaching should be individualized and should address the specific medication(s) the patient is on.

Breathing Training and Range of Motion

In addition to Frownfelter's list, the principles of breathing training should be taught in order to complement the exercise program. Breathing training consists of fundamental education and low-level physical activities that need to be mastered before the patient attempts such more conventional exercises as walking, climbing stairs, treadmill workouts, and cycling (O'Ryan, 1984b). It includes the teaching of diaphragmatic, pursed-lip breathing, as well as useful range of motion (ROM) activities that can be incorporated into daily living. The main difficulty in emphysema is the tendency of the bronchi to collapse during expiration due to their loss of elasticity and the positive intrathoracic pressure that is necessary to force air from inelastic lungs. If the lips are pursed during expiration, the pressure within the bronchi is increased because the air must be forced through the narrow opening between the lips. This encourages the bronchi to remain open during expiration, thus improving the most difficult phase of respiration. Pursed-lip expiration can be particularly important on effort and may increase the ability of the patient to perform activities which otherwise would make him severely dyspneic (Farber & Wilson, 1968).

Breathing exercises (a) help the patient get maximum ventilation from all parts of his lungs; (b) increase the strength, coordination, and efficiency of the muscles of respiration; (c) reduce the unnecessary use of accessory respiratory muscles at rest and, to a degree, while exercising at submaximal loads; (d) provide a more rhythmic and cadence type of breathing that is both physiologically and psychologically satisfying; and (e) generally make a more aesthetically acceptable type of breathing that does not call as much public attention to the patient's affliction (Farber & Wilson, 1968; O'Ryan, 1984b). The patient will need to conscientiously practice diaphragmatic, pursed-lip breathing until it becomes a fixed, spontaneous method of breathing. In learning the procedure, a patient may find it useful to implement the standard technique of mentally counting to oneself (''one thousand one, one thousand two, one thousand three, etc.'') during the inspiratory and expiratory phases of his breathing. During any physical activity performance, the patient should mentally be counting out his I:E ratios to himself.

O'Ryan (1984b) suggests that teaching ROM exercises in combination with pursed-lip breathing offers many advantages:

- It allows the patient to pursue daily activities without undue dyspnea.
- It teaches the patient to associate his daily activities with specific energy- and oxygen-conserving movements.
- It allows for more efficient and effective movement, with a greater net return of work unit gained per work unit performed.
- It allows for a transfer of the training effect.
- It serves as a warm-up prior to endurance training.
- It improves psychological outlook and morale, due to the patient's improved physical agility.

The ROM exercises illustrated in Figure 1 represent the basic abduction and adduction movements that will allow for a transfer of the training effect. These movements become more meaningful and useful to the patient when modified to fit his daily lifestyle.

Additional Educational Topics and Resources

Additional patient and family educational topics should include (Plummer, 1984)

- relaxation training,
- assistive breathing devices,
- the intricacies of blood gases,
- postural drainage,
- stretching and posture,
- work simplifications,

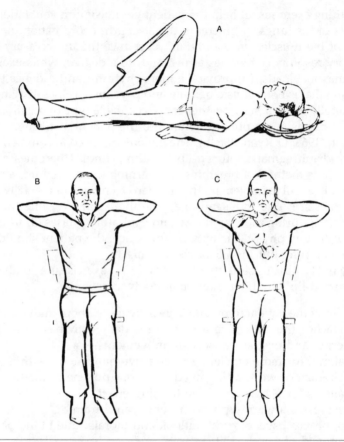

Figure 1 ROM exercises. Cardinal principles: (1) incorporate D-PLB; (2) always exhale when adducting, inhale when abducting. **A**, kneebend: patient exhales while bringing knee forward to chest and inhales while bringing knee to rest flat on table or bed. Alternate legs. **B**, modified arm raises: patient inhales while raising arms, exhales while lowering arms. **C**, elbow to knee: patient exhales while touching elbow to knee, inhales while returning to resting position. Alternate with other elbow and knee. Reproduced with permission from O'Ryan, J.A.: Pulmonary Rehabilitation Techniques, in O'Ryan, J.A., and Burns, D.G. (eds.): *Pulmonary Rehabilitation: From Hospital to Home.* Copyright © 1984 by Year Book Medical Publishers, Inc., Chicago.

- energy conservation,
- pacing,
- activities of daily living,
- use of leisure time,
- how to take one's pulse,
- sexuality,
- smoking cessation principles,
- other assorted topics to enhance coping strategies.

Films and Video Tapes

O'Ryan (1984a) provides a comprehensive evaluation of the following films in teaching a patient about lung disease:

Pulmonary Selfcare: A program for patients, by consultants Linda Doyle, R.N., M.N.C.; Eileen Hagarty, R.N., M.S.; John E. Hodgkin, M.D.; Leonard D. Hudson, M.D.; Karen Schaffran Larson, R.P.T.; Marion T. Leone, R.N.; William Walthall, R.P.T., B.S.; and William G. Zorn, R.N., M.S. Four videocassette tapes, 3/4" u-matic, 1/2" Beta, 1/2" VHS. Chicago: Encyclopedia Britannica Educational Corporation, 1980. $995 (complete set of 4 videocassettes).

The videocassette tapes include "Living with a Breathing Problem," "Learning to Breathe Better," "Clearing Your Airways," and "Building Your Strength and Endurance." The four tapes attempt to teach patients how to manage their breathing problems in simple terminology and in uncontrived, everyday settings. Accompanying the tapes is a 48-page manual for the patient and family, which contains basic information written in lay language.

PEP Series (Pulmonary Education Package), by Georgia Lung Association consultants Jane G. Gaston; Robert J. DiBenedetto, M.D.; Richard DeBorde, R.R.T., P.A.; Steve Hammong, R.R.T., P.A. Ten programs available in videocassettes or slide/tapes series. Hilton Head Island, SC Tri-Comm Productions, 1976. $600 (10 videocassettes), $350 (slide/tape series).

The topics include:

- How the Lungs Work
- What is COPD?
- Chronic Bronchitis
- What is Emphysema?
- Understanding Asthma
- Drug Therapy of COPD
- Inhalation Therapy
- Oxygen Therapy in the Home
- Breathing Exercises
- General Health Measures

I Am Joe's Lung, by National Film Board of Canada, available in videocassette. Distributed by Pyramid films.

Teaching Aids With Professional Illustrations

"Chronic Lung Disease"—an educational flipchart by Robert J. Brady Co., Bowie, MD, 20715, and "Chronic Obstructive Emphysema," reprinted from *Clinical Symposia*, Vol. 20, No. 2, 1968, and distributed by CIBA Pharmaceutical Company, Division of CIBA-Geigy Corporation, Summit, NJ.

Brochures

Brochures are also useful to patients and their families, for they are relatively inexpensive and can be kept to reexamine at later dates. The following list of brochures should be helpful.

"About Lungs and Lung Diseases"
Channing L. Bete., Co., Inc.
South Deerfield, MA 01373

"Breathing for People with Chronic Lung Disease"
Georgia Lung Association, Inc.
1383 Spring Street, N.W.
Atlanta, GA 30309

"Living at Home with: COPD"
Travenol Laboratories, Inc.
Respiratory Homecare
One Baxter Parkway
Deerfield, IL 60015

"Save Your Breath!"
Bolhringer Ingelheim Ltd.
Ridgefield, CT 06877

"The Do's and Don't's of Walking"
Breon Laboratories Inc.
90 Park Avenue
New York, NY 10016

Numerous educational brochures (catalog is available) can be ordered from the American Lung Association (or local affiliate), 1740 Broadway, New York, NY 10019.

"Clearing the Air" and "Calling it Quits"
Officer of Cancer Communications
National Cancer Institute
Building 31, Room 10A29
Bethesda, MD 20205

Educational Manuals include:

Staff Manual for Teaching Patients About Chronic Obstructive
Pulmonary Diseases, 1982 edition.
American Hospital Association

840 North Lake Shore Drive
Chicago, IL 60611

Respiratory Rehabilitation: A Comprehensive Approach. Edited by: John
E. Hodgkins, M.D.; Eileen G. Zorn, R.N., M.S. and Glen N. Gee, R.R.T.
Distributed through the courtesy of Parke-Davis Pharmaceuticals.

Better Living and Breathing: A Manual for Patients
Pulmonary Division
University of California, San Diego
The C.V. Mosby Co.
11830 Westline Industrial Drive
St. Louis, MO 63141

Assessing patient readiness, establishing learning objectives, setting pri-
orities, coordinating the multidisciplinary educational team, selecting
resources, and implementing strategies to encourage patient education
and to promote learning are all essential ingredients for an effective educational program. However, in the final analysis, it is the patient who must
assume responsibility for his or her own health care. Yet, learning abilities among patients are often subtly impaired. This can be remedied by
estimating the patient's learning skills and adjusting the program to the
patient's ability, and requiring the patient to demonstrate new knowledge and skills before progressing further. The patient must be viewed
in terms of the personal and environmental assets at his or her disposal.
These include family and social support, potential employment skills,
employment opportunities, and community resources. These all need to
be evaluated and mobilized for practical help to the patient and to bolster his or her motivation (American Thoracic Society, 1982).

Conclusion

The physiological, psychological, and educational benefits of pulmonary
rehabilitation have been discussed in this chapter. However, there are
those who continue to question the financial worth of such a program.
They shouldn't: Persons suffering from COPD frequently require
hospitalization for treatment of recurrent lung infections and exacerbations of symptoms. Hospitalizations result in ever-increasing medical
costs, which are incurred by third-party payers such as Blue Cross and
Blue Shield, Medicare and Medicaid, but which eventually are borne by
the community—and the nation as a whole—in the form of increased medical care expenditure (MacDonnell, 1983).

Sahn, Nett and Petty (1980) have shown that the frequency of admis-
sions to the hospital because of exacerbations of the symptoms of COPD

may be lessened by preventive health care measures. One such preventive health measure is pulmonary rehabilitation. The major goal of pulmonary rehabilitation is to provide the patient with the proper information, education, psychological support, exercise guidelines, and medical care to effectively reduce the need for repeated hospitalizations.

References

American College of Sports Medicine. (1980). *Guidelines for graded exercise testing and exercise prescription* (2nd ed.). Philadelphia: Lea and Febiger.

American Thoracic Society-Medical Section of the American Lung Association. (1982). In C.W. Bell et al. (Eds.), *Home care and rehabilitation in respiratory medicine*. Philadelphia: J.B. Lippincott.

Barach, A.L., Bickerman, H.A., & Beck, G.J. (1972). Advances in the treatment of nontuberculous pulmonary disease. *Bulletin of the New York Academy of Medicine, 28*, 353.

Beck, A.T. (1972). Measuring depression: The depression inventory. In T. Williams, M. Katz, & J. Shields (Eds.), *Recent advances in the psychobiology of the depressive illness*. Washington, DC: U.S. Government Printing Office.

Bell, C.W. (1980). Pulmonary rehabilitation and exercise testing. In P.K. Wilson, C.W. Bell, & A.C. Norton (Eds.), *Rehabilitation of the heart and lungs* (pp. 15-34). Fullerton, CA: Beckman Instruments.

Belman, J.J., & Wasserman, K. (1982). *Respiratory Care, 27*, 724-731.

Blodgett, D. (1982). Relaxation techniques. In C.W. Bell et al. (Eds.), *Home care and rehabilitation in respiratory medicine*. Philadelphia: J.B. Lippincott.

Brown, S.R., Fregosi, R., & Reddan, W. (1982). Exercise training in patients with COPD. *Chronic Obstructive Pulmonary Disease, 71*, 163-173.

Butts, J.R. (1981). Pulmonary rehabilitation through exercise and education. *CVP, 13*(2), 17-21, 60-61.

Cotes, J.E., & Gilson, J.C. (1956). Effect of oxygen on exercise ability in chronic respiratory insufficiency: Use of portable apparatus. *Lancet, 1*, 872-876.

Dudley, D.L. (1980). Psychological concomitants to rehabilitation in chronic obstructive pulmonary disease: I. Pyschosocial and psychological considerations. *Chest, 77*, 413-420.

Farber, S.M., & Wilson, R.H. (1968). Chronic obstructive emphysema. *Clinical Symposia, 20*, 35-69.

Frownfelter, D.L. (1979a). Pulmonary rehabilitation. In D.L. Frownfelter (Ed.), *Chest physical therapy and pulmonary rehabilitation: An interdisciplinary approach* (pp. 13-34). Chicago: Year Book Medical Publishers.

Frownfelter, D.L. (1979b). Relaxation principles and techniques. In D.L. Frownfelter (Ed.), *Chest physical therapy and pulmonary rehabilitation: An interdisplinary approach*. Chicago: Year Book Medical Publishers.

Gartner, A.J., & Riessman, F. (1982). Self-help and mental health. *Hospital Community Psychiatry*, **33**, 631-635.

Holliday, J.E. (1984). Biofeedback. In J.A. O'Ryan & D.G. Burns (Eds.), *Pulmonary rehabilitation: From hospital to home* (pp. 85-111). Chicago: Year Book Medical Publishers.

Holliday, J.E., & Munz, D. (1978). Changes in locus of control due to biofeedback. In *Proceedings of the Ninth Annual Meeting of the Biofeedback Society of America*. Alberquerque, N.M.

Ledwidge, B. (1980). Run for your mind: Aerobic exercise as a means of alleviating anxiety and depression. *Canadian Journal of Behavioral Science*, **12**, 2-12.

MacDonnell, R.J. (1983). The pulmonary rehabilitation maze. *Respiratory Care*, **28**, 180-190.

Meissner, J.R. (1980). Semantic diffferential scales for assessing patients' feelings. *Nursing 80*, **2**, 70-71.

Miller, W.F., Taylor, H.F., & Pierce, A.K. (1963). Rehabilitation of the disabled patient with chronic bronchitis and pulmonary emphysema. *American Journal of Public Health*, **53**(Suppl. 3), 18.

O'Ryan, J.A. (1984a). Audiovisuals and print media: aids and organizations. In J.A. O'Ryan & D.G. Burns (Eds.), *Pulmonary rehabilitation: From hospital to home*. Chicago: Year Book Medical Publishers.

O'Ryan, J.A. (1984b). Pulmonary rehabilitation techniques. In J.A. O'Ryan & D.C. Burns (Eds.) *Pulmonary rehabilitation: From hospital to home* (pp. 64-81). Chicago: Year book Medical Publishers.

Paez, P.N., Phillipson, E.A., & Massangkay, M. (1967). The physiologic basis of training patients with emphysema. *American Review of Respiratory Diseases*, **95**, 944-953.

Petty, T.L., & Nelt, L.M. (1978). Pulmonary rehabilitation. *Continuing Education*, **9**, 28-39.

Plummer, J.K. (1984). Psychological factors in pulmonary rehabilitation. In J.A. O'Ryan & D.G. Burns (Eds.), *Pulmonary rehabilitation: From hospital to home* (pp. 146-166). Chicago: Year Book Medical Publishers.

Sahn, S., Nett, L., & Petty, T. (1980). Ten year follow-up of a comprehensive rehabilitation program for COPD. *Chest*, **77**, 311-314.

Seiler, L.H. (1979). *Final report: The fifteen-month patient education study*. New York: American Lung Association.

Shephard, R.J. (1976). Exercise and chronic obstructive lung disease. *Exercise Sport and Science Review*, **4**, 263-296.

Spielberg, J. (1968). *State-trait anxiety inventory*. Consulting Psychologists Press.

University of Washington, Department of Health Services. (1978). *Sickness impact profile*. Seattle: University of Washington Press.

Vyas, M.N., Banister, E.W., & Morton, J.W. (1971). Response to exercise in patients with chronic airway obstruction: II. Effects of breathing 40% oxygen. *American Review of Respiratory Diseases*, **103**, 401-412.

Woolf, C.R., & Swero, J.T. (1969). Alterations in lung mechanics and gas exchange following training in chronic obstructive lung disease. *Diseases of Chest*, **55**, 37.

Zung, C.W. (1965). Zung depression inventory. *Archives of General Psychiatry*, **12**, 63-70.